PERSONALIZED MEDICINE

PERSONALIZED MEDICINE
Regaining and
Maintaining Health

Dr. Jean-Claude Lapraz and
Marie-Laure de Clermont-Tonnerre

AEON

Aeon Books Ltd
12 New College Parade Finchley Road
London NW3 5EP

British Library Cataloguing in Publication Data

A C.I.P. for this book is available from the British Library

ISBN-13: 978-1-91280-787-1

Typeset by Medlar Publishing Solutions Pvt Ltd, India

www.aeonbooks.co.uk

CONTENTS

PREFACE TO THE ENGLISH-LANGUAGE EDITION

Endobiogeny is a term doubtless unfamiliar to most English-speakers, even those with a particular interest in 'integrative' approaches to physiology and medicine. *Personalized Medicine* is the first English-language introduction to this developing science, written jointly by its foremost living exponent—Dr. Jean-Claude Lapraz—and by a journalist who was also his patient—Marie-Laure de Clermont-Tonnerre. It is aimed both at the general public and at members of the health professions.

What is there about the approach of Dr. Lapraz and his former colleague, Dr. Christian Duraffourd, that offers hope to patients such as Marie-Laure, who suffer from serious, chronic and apparently incurable conditions? These two doctors developed a diagnostic method that, while being rooted in modern science, allows an insight into the true causes of imbalance and disease in a patient; far from being backward-looking, it uses a systems approach that is in line with the most modern scientific thinking. The choice of medicinal plants as therapeutic agents fits perfectly with this approach, as *Personalized Medicine* explains. The book explains Endobiogenic principles and methods, including the modelling system known as the Biology of Functions, and is full of remarkable case histories that attest to the efficacy of this approach.

According to Dr. Lapraz, the method of Endobiogeny is three-fold: listening to the patient, examining them carefully, and analysing their bloodwork using the Biology of Functions. For patient and practitioner alike, this offers a rich experience. For the patient, being heard—and believed—is validating, and brings insights. There is a call for you to be empowered, to step into a place of healing and wellness. This is an active pursuit of health that requires your participation at every step of the journey. For the care-provider, empowerment comes from clarity of diagnosis and confidence in prescribing personalized care. Finally, medicine returns to art of wellness!

Originating in France, Endobiogeny has now been taught to health practitioners in a number of countries, as outlined in chapter 7. It has been for us a great pleasure to work alongside Dr. Lapraz in diffusing the knowledge of Endobiogeny throughout the world. I (Kamyar Hedayat) have, since 2010, with Dr. Lapraz developed international training programmes in Endobiogenic medicine. Through our research and educational company SBRG, we have created a certification program to ensure the highest level of training in the authentic vision of Endobiogeny as taught by Drs. Duraffourd and Lapraz. In addition, Dr. Lapraz and I have been active in clinical research, the first ever three-volume textbook, and a handbook of Endobiogenic Medicine for doctors in practice (Elsevier, 2019). Now more than ever, physicians are being trained in Endobiogeny to meet the growing interest of patients for participatory medicine that is at once scientific and humanistic.

In the United Kingdom, from 1990 to 2010, I (Colin Nicholls) organized a series of training seminars in Endobiogeny for medical herbalists and health professionals, led originally by Dr. Lapraz and more recently by Dr. Hedayat. As a former Program Leader of the BSc and MSc Herbal Medicine practitioner training programs at Middlesex University, and one of a small group of medical herbalists in the UK who have SBRG certification in foundational Endobiogeny concepts, I am committed, together with my colleagues, to making this revolutionary medical approach more available both to the general public and to health professionals in the UK. Projects currently under development include an entry-level Endobiogenic program for GPs and other medical professionals.

We hope that *Personalized Medicine*, exploring Endobiogeny as it does from a dual perspective, will inspire both patients and practitioners in the English-speaking world to re-examine the whole concept of appropriate medical practice, and to adopt Endobiogenic philosophy as central both to the maintenance of their own health and to the health-care that they offer to others.

Colin Nicholls
President, Endobiogenic Medicine Society (UK)
www.endobio.org.uk

Kamyar M. Hedayat, MD
President, American Society of Endobiogenic
Medicine and Integrative Physiology
www.asemip.org
Co-President, Systems Biology Research Group
Medical Director, Full Spectrum Health: An Endobiogeny
Medical Center
Chicago, Illinois, USA

It was in France a lifetime ago that I encountered herbal medicine for the first time, so my meeting with Dr. Jean-Claude Lapraz, and later studying and working with him in Paris, felt like coming home after my long pathways of study here in England and many else-wheres. I felt privileged, therefore, to be asked to undertake the transla-tion of *La Médicine Personnalisée* which had been translated already into Lithuanian by a professional translator, which I cannot claim to be.

The year or so I spent on the project coincided with my studying in that country. Much of the work was undertaken as I crossed the Baltic by ship or the plains of Europe by various means. My destination the city of Kaunas, my purpose of travel was to the seminars given there by Dr Kamyar Hedayat. His outstanding teaching and clinical instruc-tion will, I hope, have managed to iron out any waves and eddies cre-ated by my divers modes of transport. It was a most happy experience in that most hospitable Baltic country and I must thank Nicolas Ortiz, co–founder of the Endobiogenic Society of Lithuania (Endobiogenikos Draugija), for his encouragement and financial support of my project to bring the extraordinary developments in herbal medicine made by Dr Lapraz into English. He wishes to acknowledge the collaborative support of his two brothers towards the whole Endobiogenic initiative.

PREFACE TO THE SECOND EDITION

More than six years have passed since the first edition of this book appeared in 2011, published by Odile Jacob. During this time, a number of research projects have been conducted, both in France and overseas, to evaluate the soundness and efficacy of the Endobiogenic approach in patients. These consist in:

- Clinical studies into the effects of this approach applied to those with a wide range of illnesses as well as subjects in good health leading to a broader understanding of presenting symptoms.
- Analysis of findings provided by the biology of functions in daily practice correlated with clinical findings.
- Ongoing research from hospital, retrospective as well as prospective, within various departments of medicine: cardiology, endocrinology, metabolic disorders, gynaecology, along with novel techniques for evaluating stress.
- Setting up of training courses and seminars for medical personnel in various countries: England, USA (under the auspices of ASEMIP, SBRG), France, (SIMEPI) Lithuania (EMD Lithuanian Society of Endobiogeny), Mexico (SoMeFic Mexican Society of Endobiogeny) and the

creation in France of an Institute of Endobiogeny (contact:institut. endobiogenie@gmail.com)

- The publication in scientific journals on the endobiogenic approach and the biology of functions:
Endobiogeny: a global approach to systems biology (part 1 of 2). Lapraz JC, Hedayat KM. *Glob Adv Health Med.* 2013 Jan;2(1):64–78. doi: 10.7453/gahmj.2013.2.1.011. Review. PMID: 24381827 Endobiogeny: a global approach to systems biology (part 2 of 2). Lapraz JC, Hedayat KM, Pauly P. *Glob Adv Health Med.* 2013 Mar;2(2):32–44. doi: 10.7453/gahmj.2013.013. Review. PMID: 24416662. A novel use of biomarkers in the modeling of cancer activity based on the theory of endobiogeny. Buehning LJ, Hedayat KM, Sachdeva A, Golshan S, Lapraz JC. *Glob Adv Health Med.* 2014 Jul;3(4):55–60. doi: 10.7453/gahmj.2013.041. PMID: 25105079. Genito-Thyroid Index: A Global Systems Approach to the Neutrophil-to-Lymphocyte Ratio According to the Theory of Endobiogeny Applied to Ambulatory Patients with Chronic Heart Failure. Kamyar M. Hedayat, Benjamin M. Schuff, Jean-Claude Lapraz, Tiffany Barsotti, Shahrokh Golshan, Suzi Hong, Barry H. Greenberg, and Paul J. Mills. *J Cardiol Clin Res.* 5(1): 1091 (2017).

- Other publications:
- *Plantes médicinales, Phytothérapie Clinique Intégrative et Médecine Endobiogénique* Lavoisier 2017, a collective work under the direction of doctors JC Lapraz et A. Carillon with doctors JC Charrié, K. Hedayat and doctors in pharmacy B. Chastel, C. Cieur, P. Combe, M. Damak, C. Saigne-Soulard. chapters on phytotherapy and pharmacy, are succeeded by 45 detailed monographs on medicinal plants. This original work rests on a new approach to the use of these plants, putting the patient at the centre of diagnostic and therapeutic thought and procedures. This approach allows plants to be use in an integrative and personalised manner in relying on both traditional knowledge and the findings of modern pharmacology. Because of the complexity of the elements which make them up and with their specific actions, medicinal plants are best used therapeutically in disturbances of physiology and so may provide a first line of treatment providing they are prescribed according to medical disciplines. Endobiogenic medicine provides a thoughtful and original method for bringing the disturbances of the neuro–endocrine systems that direct the health of living beings. It helps the physician identify them and allows

treatment that regulates physiology where medicinal plants play a primary role in helping the individual recover the state of health that preceded the illness.

- *Les clés de l'alimentation anti-cancer, anti-inflammatoire, anti-infectieuse, anti maladie auto-immune* Dr. JC Charrié, Maryse Groussard & Sophie Bartczak. Paris 2012; *Se soigner toute l'année au naturel* Dr. JC Charrié et Marie-Laure de Clermont-Tonnerre. Editions Prat Paris 2015; *En bonne santé toute l'année: 20 cures alimentaires naturelles et efficaces* Dr. JC Charrié et Marie-Laure de Clermont–Tonnerre Editions Terre-vivante Paris 2017.

- The results provided by these and other works in preparation all tend to confirm the validity of the theory behind the endobiogenic approach toward the patient, fully supporting the substance of the 'Personalised Medicine', and show the immense possibilities for preventative and curative treatments afforded by integrative clinical phytotherapy. We would hope that those in charge of public health would give these research findings the attention they deserve and allow scientifically validated therapies to enter into the medical culture and the training of doctors and pharmacists so that all patients may benefit from personalised medicine.

Dr. J.-C. Lapraz

FOREWORD

This book is intended for both the general public and for the medical community. It was born out of the encounter between a physician and his journalist patient.

For the physician, this book answers a need to present to the world the fruits of his 40 years of private and hospital practice. His principal aim has been to develop a true terrain-based medicine, one that is both preventative and curative. Working with French and foreign colleagues, the aim has always been to treat each individual patient as a whole person.

For the journalist, novel answers were given to all her questions about illness and health. They emerged during the course of writing these pages as well as during the journey she took during these consultations. She will invite you into the confidential heart of medical consultations with other patients where you can be the fly on the wall. None of the patients objected to her presence, which she took as a sign of their respect for Dr. Lapraz, and their desire to share what they themselves had discovered. You will hear them speak in their own words, and as they talk about themselves, they might well be speaking for you.

To all those who are tired of swallowing antibiotics, steroids, anti-inflammatory medicines, beta blockers, anticoagulants, or painkillers, at the first sign of illness, yet still suffer a relapse. What can one do when treatments fail to work or, worse still, cause further problems? What hope is there for those suffering from serious illness?

This book offers a new medical vision that treats each person as an integrated whole and stands in contrast to modern medical practice—so often standardized and excessively specialized—which focuses on symptoms and dissociates the disease from the patient. Personalized Medicine presents a new and different approach to the patient, the disease and the treatment.

This original integrative concept, called Endobiogeny, offers the key to a novel approach to health, both for medical care and prevention, and also for support when the patient has to undergo conventional chemical treatments.

This new personalized medical approach is truly predictive, and in treating the individual as a whole person is not hostile to any medical practice. It is fully at home in daily medical practice, fully in accord with all the rules that govern the art and science of medicine. Doctors in many countries now practice Endobiogeny: to prevent, to treat and to cure. What kind of healthcare do we want for tomorrow? Don't we all deserve medical care that respects our specificity and our uniqueness, a form of medicine that is truly preventative and that offers treatment that causes the least harm?

A patient like you: why this book can answer your questions about your health

We all have questions about the treatments we receive! Perhaps like many of you, someone in my close circle of friends is suffering from serious illness and I am sorry to have to say that the care provided for her and the powerful synthetic drugs she has been prescribed are no longer much help anymore. It is already too late. This is why I have so many questions particularly about prevention. Could we not have done something sooner? What factors, what physiological processes caused this person to develop this particular disease, which has caused her so much suffering? In France, we have screening programs for early detection such as mammograms, ultrasound and biopsies, but nothing is done for prevention. But we need a comprehensive approach to the patient that will lead to an effective understanding of the imbalances at work in the body that will, if unchecked, lead to disease.

I had been asking myself if disease happens to us by "chance" or is it perhaps just the name we give to our ignorance? Should we be fatalistic, or should we be able take care of ourselves and our own health? Are there unfavorable terrains that allowing one disease or another to take hold? Should we get to know our physiological strengths and weaknesses so as to recognize any imbalances and that way take better care of ourselves?

I was looking for answers to my questions on the causes of disease, the treatments available (whether allopathy, homeopathy or herbal medicine), and the part played by the patient in his or her pathology, together with the notion of cure. Is healing only about making symptoms disappear? Or should we go deeper and try to treat the root causes of the illness? However, who is capable of this in the medical system practiced in France and more generally in the West? There is no shortage of complementary or alternative modalities, which claim to be holistic. They purport to offer a comprehensive approach to disease and have become very popular, but there is also a growing apprehension about the quality of care offered by practitioners of these so-called alternative medical practices. They claim to treat the whole patient and not just the disease. Good idea, but how can one be sure that these practitioners are competent to make a critical and personalized diagnosis? Without formal medical training how can we be certain that they will not endanger patients by failing to fully understand the consequences of the treatments they prescribe?

Neither is there any shortage of ready-made dietary advice and anecdotal recommendations. Then there are all kind of diets, miracle drinks, and plants that are promoted in books and magazines as cures for everything. Who can believe in all these more or less miraculous promises made in this period of alarming progression of certain diseases? It would be nice to think that eating more chocolate, going to the gym, drinking pomegranate juice, or taking turmeric would protect me from all manner of diseases, but I was looking for a wide-ranging, more informed medical answer that might offer us, the patients new insights.

I had begun to doubt the ability of modern medicine to treat me as a whole person, without asking me to take unwarranted risks. This fear is stirred up by recent scandals on the harmfulness of certain medicinal products such as Acomplia [Rimonabant],[1] Mediator [Benfluorex][2] and Vioxx [Rofecoxib].[3] As they have been withdrawn from sale, I am not the only one to have lost confidence.

A crisis of confidence

This crisis of confidence in our medical system is part of a more general challenge and is of the same order that calls into question our financial institutions and economic structures, which are currently out of control. We have entered an age of anxiety in which the certainties of the past cannot be taken for granted anymore, an age in which we have to question everything.

Patients are often left to face their problems on their own. Gloomy statistics about the escalation of cancers remind us of the limits and sometimes the helplessness of modern medicine. Cancer is now likely to affect one in two men and one in three women during their lifetime. In his last book, *Les Combats de la vie: mieux que guérir, prévenir* (*"The Fight For Life: Prevention Is Better Than Treatment"*), Professor Luc Montagnier, winner of the 2008 Nobel Prize for Medicine, states: "Here, [in France], too many young adults die prematurely from cancer[4] or heart attacks, and diseases of the nervous system as well as disabling joint conditions are on the increase as we are all living longer."

Disturbing figures published in the United States reveal the scale of the iatrogenic effect and how medicinal products claim a significant number of lives by their toxicity.[5] This is unsettling if one stops to think that France is the world's largest consumer of antibiotics, antidepressants, and sedatives.

Do you experience a feeling of powerlessness?

We all feel powerless when we don't understand what is happening to us and have to put up with disabling symptoms, a feeling made worse when we feel that those with medical knowledge treat us like children. A poorly chosen remark when we are feeling vulnerable can make us distraught or leave us with unanswered questions. Sometimes, doctors hurriedly inform us in a tone that is terse and which brooks no discussion, about possible troubles that we may have to face. In blunt medical terminology, they deliver us a list of standardized procedures that we shall have to undergo: "We are going to lower your cholesterol ... We will deal with the virus ... We will bombard the cancer cell ... You just need to take these medicinal products." We are sometimes treated with the same standard protocol as if we were mere numbers. The current medical approach has dug a ditch between the patients and their disease. It implies that the disease belongs to them rather than their patients, the exclusive property of those specialized in the art.

This is what we can expect if we are unfortunate enough to develop cancer or some other serious disease. Welcome to the world we have allowed to take root: a world often cold, medicalized, technical, and sometimes dehumanized; a world where it is difficult to get hold of the simplest item of information. A world you have to wait for hours to be hastily examined, where doctors have one eye on the patient and one eye on the clock. Besides the hurried nature of the examination, with clinicians having no time to listen to the patient, the modern healthcare system presents the distraught patient with other problems, such as prescriptions written in a state of urgency, leading inevitably to inappropriate prescriptions, excessive specialization which leads to the patient being treated as if fragmented into parts, with the pieces never being put back together again. This complete absence of synthesis fails to respect the complexity and the interrelatedness of everything at work in the body and gives no consideration to the uniqueness of each person's terrain; it treats the patient and the disease as if they were separate entities.

Is this the kind of medicine we want?

But what can doctors do when faced with a healthcare system governed by powerful economic forces which requires them to prescribe harmful and costly medicinal products to all their patients, when they know that only a small fraction of them really need them? Shouldn't they be permitted to offer less harmful treatments that are less costly, and better adapted to the physiology of their patients for whom powerful medication is not strictly necessary? In the United States, a country we often look to, they have seen a surge in demand for customized healthcare of a call for the use of less toxic treatments.

Surely it would be in the patient's best interest to have doctors take a critical look at their work and, without abandoning modern scientific methods, come up with some original solutions, and adopt a fresh approach. From my own investigations and research into healthcare options, I came across a group of French doctors associated with Doctor Jean-Claude Lapraz who, in spite of having gone through the mill of medical school, have had the courage to think outside the box. For the most part, they had worked in hospital departments so their calling into question the status quo and their search for fresh solutions derive from experience at the coalface of modern medical practice. This is what motivated me to spend time with them, to observe and try to understand their original and innovative ideas, so that I could spread the word about a new approach to medicine that put the patient back at the heart of the system.

Their concrete results in terms of prevention, relief, or improvement of serious disease, and the stabilization or cure of chronic diseases fired me up with enthusiasm to sit in on their medical consultations as an observer, to attend their professional seminars, courses and international research projects. I became convinced of the importance of testifying as to what I leaned. They strive always to prescribe the safest effective treatments, which no doubt explains why their waiting rooms are never empty.

Sharing in medical consultations: a privilege

The other voice in this book is therefore mine, that of a patient, like you, a voice that will try to answer the questions you might have. I spent a whole year with Dr. Lapraz, I sat in on numerous consultations and collected the testimony of patients, always with their full consent. As a silent witness, I saw very intimate and often distressing situations unfold before my eyes. Patients did not seem inhibited as they confided in him during the consultation, in spite of my presence. Dr. Lapraz's carefully aimed questions drew them out and encouraged them to reveal inner conflicts and it seemed to me that taking responsibility for their health and their account of their illness being taken seriously has changed the way they see themselves, and this eased their suffering. In a word, they were won over.

Dr. Lapraz's approach is first to listen at length to his patients, then examine them carefully, taking the time to interpret what he found and then explaining his conclusions clearly and to the point, and then guiding and supporting them through their illness once the diagnosis has been made. This is how he and his colleagues work, day in, day out, he takes care of the troubles that afflict his fellow human beings. This is the story of how, from 9 o'clock in the morning until very late in the evening, he sees patients who are full of hope having been brought to him by word-of-mouth. People from all walks of life: farmers, actors and teachers rubbing shoulders with politicians and nuns, workers and their bosses, all coming to Paris for an appointment. Nothing would make them miss their appointment with this doctor who sees his patients as a whole person and takes personal interest in their treatment, constantly checking the precise status of their terrain. So many afflictions, life stories, human voices, which could be mine, or could be yours.

I have sat in on many of these consultations, often with curiosity and the desire to understand, with wonderment and sometimes with distress, but also with the fear of being confronted with serious illness, and having to look those who are suffering in the eye. Dr. Lapraz is the same attentive, calm, and empathic self for all his patients. Never a word of impatience, never glancing at his watch. Here, there is no sense of time; it is devoted to others, a time for humanity. His very precise, often unexpected, questions, his powers of observation, his kindness which invites the patients to say the inexpressible, to cry, to find release. He dedicates these consultations to listening to others so they become an oasis of reassurance where fears can be overcome and self–worth be restored, given a quality of attention rare in a society in which nobody hears you anymore.

In this book, I want to talk about those who came to unburden them-selves, about the often courageous way they tackled their illness. For all that, I haven't abandoned my critical faculties and can tell the difference between the placebo effect of soothing words and the hard facts of real results obtained by the recovery sick patients, or preventative measures by those in good health. It took me a long time to fully understand the subtlety and complexity of such demanding medicine that aims for an understanding of the integrity and uniqueness of each patient as a whole person.

My reservations as a journalist

Before embarking on this adventure, I wanted to learn more about this doctor whose methods differ so from those of his colleagues. In my search, I came across the book written by one of his American patients, Carol Silverander from Santa Barbara, (see Chapter 9 "Carol's Case: Metastatic Breast Cancer"). This opened up entirely new prospects. I ordered it and read it within a few days with great interest. The cover shows a smiling woman, who seems to emanate boundless energy and drive. The title is written in big letters, *With the Help of Our Friends from France. Stabilizing and Living with Advanced Breast Cancer*. It had been a great success in the United States when first published in 2005, and attracted a huge following; TV interviews and articles followed. The second edition, published in 2007, was written, after all, by a patient who had been told in 1999 that she probably had just 2 more years to live.

It was a moving story: the battle of a woman who wanted to live with dignity and courage, and who refused to allow fear to take possession of her spirit. Throughout the book, she talks in detail about the positive impact that the medical approach of Dr. Jean-Claude Lapraz and his colleague Dr. Christian Duraffourd had on her disease. In collaboration with her American oncologist, they had established very precise strategies to stabilize her illness, which was already very advanced.

For those patients suffering from cancer, I could see, following the thread of consultations, how this doctor was attempting to give them new insights into the mechanisms at work in their bodies, which were the source of their disease. You could also follow how he sought to stabilize or care for these patients, who had been weakened by the powerful treatments given by their oncologists. With other diseases, or with a view to prevention, I was very impressed by the accuracy of the diagnosis, which he came to by a meticulous and personalized consultation, and corroborated with biological criteria which appeared to represent a real step forward for patients (see Chapter 3 "A True Terrain-Based Medicine: New Hope for Patients").

I was also impressed by the care he took, once the diagnosis had been made, to formulate the least toxic treatment. I notice that he was at pains to support the natural defenses of the body rather than trying at all costs to bolster them up with something invasive. I wondered why such treatment is not more freely available.

The book you are currently holding followed lengthy and lively discussions between this doctor and me, which continued unabated during the writing period. On the one hand, Dr. Lapraz sought to convince me of the need for a more personalized medicine with effective, highly targeted treatments that carried the least risk of harm. On the other, there is me, the skeptical journalist, or perhaps someone simply not ready to embrace such innovative change, and resistant to radical ideas. Faced with my doubts and my questions, he sought to be as transparent as possible and arranged for me to interview those patients I wanted to meet on my own. My concerns were also alleviated when I came to appreciate the extent to which he worked with other colleagues (oncologists, dermatologists, pediatricians, surgeons, and others) in a spirit of true scientific collaboration, for the greater benefit of his patients.

Over the course of many months, I interviewed his patients, some of whom he had followed-up for more than 30 years. Some of them were doctors themselves who, once they became ill, were eager to seek this doctor's advice. I sought the opinions of both his collaborators and detractors and so, little by little, I was able to come to my own conclusions. Everything in this book is therefore the fruit of these enquiries and the exchanges that took place between Doctor Lapraz and I, a process of endless questioning about the best way to look after ourselves.

When I came to the end of these inquiries, I was left wondering why this doctor who draws so many patients does not attract more attention within our medical system in France. By contrast, several foreign medical authorities have become involved, following the great interest shown by many French, American, Mexican, Tunisian and Chinese doctors (see Chapter 7 "The Growing International Influence of Clinical Phytotherapy").[6] Why did French doctors have to go to the United States, Mexico, or China to train colleagues in other countries and see their ideas adopted by medical authorities over there? Shouldn't we make a serious appraisal of this approach in French hospitals, and to focus on means of prevention based upon these methods?

A book written for you

Always willing to answer my questions, when I first made the proposal to Dr. Jean-Claude Lapraz that we write a book together, he accepted with enthusiasm. You will find his impassioned answers to my questions, always fascinating, in the chapters that follow. His vision of a more integrative approach, sitting comfortably with medicine as it is currently practiced in France, would allow us to achieve a better way to prevent and treat, restore hope, and offer real care to the sick, whether affected by simple conditions or more serious diseases. This new kind of medicine, developed from and validated by many years of practice, is the foundational resource for an integrative method and has been adopted by numerous doctors in France and abroad.

It would offer a better understanding of today's major health issues such as raised cholesterol, diabetes and other diseases of civilization and a critical assessment of the screening, treatment and prevention of cancer and degenerative diseases. It would provide us with useful clues about disease relapse and treatment failure, inappropriate prescribing and drug-induced illnesses.

You may recognize your own situation or that of your loved ones through the examples presented here. This book may also give you better resources for coping with your chronic ailments and give you a better understanding of those diseases which most frighten us. I also hope readers will benefit from the information provided, and help them put the right questions to their own doctors.

Now, I invite you to follow me. You will have the privilege to eavesdrop, in the most intimate way, to these consultations which offer a roadmap for this new kind of medicine.

CHAPTER ONE

The doctor takes up the story: early sense of fulfillment as a junior doctor

In 1970, at the age of 28, as soon as I had finished my studies at the Faculty of Medicine in Paris, and just released from military service, I started in practice as a general practitioner in the 15th arrondissement of Paris.

The experience of my years of training on the wards, coupled with expertise acquired from nights on call at the Resuscitation Unit of the Paris hospital system accustomed me to have to deal with serious cases, with the need to act quickly when caring for a dying patient, to administer overpowering antispasmodics to those in agony. With confidence in the scientific knowledge gained from my teachers, I decided to devote myself to the practice of general medicine.

Yet, only a few years earlier, I had been tempted to specialize in psychiatry when, as a young trainee at the Salpêtrière Hospital, I had been in awe of the expertise of the big names in neuropsychiatry, of their ability to come to very precise diagnoses, based on a handful of symptoms, on diseases that affected the core of a patient's humanity, their spirit. But I realized very quickly that the psychiatric approach to mental illness was woefully incomplete. It made a radical dissociation between what the patients had to say—their stories, phobias, anguish and delusions—and their bodily experiences. At no time was their

1

experience considered worthy of being taken into account in making the diagnosis, and even less in the treatment. This dissociation troubled me and seemed somewhat schizophrenic, as if there were no concord between spirit and matter.

Convinced that one cannot be a doctor without having a deep knowledge of human anatomy, I began my hospital training with a six-month stint at Cochin Hospital within the Department of Morbid Anatomy, followed by pediatrics, gynecology, gastroenterology, neurology, medical emergencies, and surgery at various hospitals in Paris. Here again, what caught my attention in every case, was a new kind of separation, similar in many ways to what I had seen in psychiatry. The notion of spirit was set aside and held to be of no account. The body was considered only in terms of histological structures, receptors, and biological functions. It was totally removed from the reality of the living being, imbued with emotions, sensibilities, joys and sorrows. Another instance of alienation was the inability or unwillingness to work towards a synthesis allowing us to understand the human being in his or her globality of being made of matter and spirit.

After 7 years of study, I came to realize that however remarkable our professors may have been in teaching their specialty, they rarely envisioned the whole person within the disease they were discussing. And yet, it was clear to me that every human body operates as a unique living entity, and for this reason, if we cannot limit ourselves by dissecting it into its parts without reintegrating them into a unified organism.

I think it was this realization that stopped me enrolling in the internship examination. This is the mandatory pathway for those wishing to specialize in a body system or organ, or a disease, a path followed by many of my colleagues, but I was deeply interested in treating the patient in their entirety. I can well understand that, given the complexity of the human being, the appeal of specialization and devoting your efforts to identifying genes or uncovering the biochemical basis of certain disorders. I appreciate the importance of understanding the role that cellular mechanisms play in the expression of disease. But my choice was made: I would become a general practitioner.

Setting up consulting rooms and starting out in general practice in Paris was never easy. That is why as a fallback, while working during the day with my first patients, I decided to be on call for the night shifts for the 7th and 15th arrondissement and also for a medical emergency team.

You have to act fast when you work in Emergency. Without effective and speedy action, the patient will surely die. It is in these most urgent cases, such as cardiac arrest, ectopic pregnancy, peritonitis and the like, where the tremendous advances of modern medicine save lives. In such circumstances, the body is in urgent need of external intervention as its capacity for self-healing has been overwhelmed and so needs massive support for failing organs. With all the means at his disposal, the doctor must decide immediately on what kind of hospital care or surgery to provide.

This was in the 1970s, 40 years ago! With all the zeal and conviction of a passionate young doctor, I tried to apply to my patients by day the successful therapeutic methods observed at the various hospitals and Resuscitation Units where I had worked. By day, the bread-and-butter cases of general practice paraded through my consulting room: infections of the ear, nose and throat, asthma, eczema, back pain for which I prescribed antibiotics, cortisone, anti-inflammatory medicines and painkillers, as I had been taught. My patients were satisfied, their pain subsided, their symptoms went away. Goodbye migraine, diarrhea, shortness of breath, hemorrhaging, inflamed tonsils and eczema. I felt that I was fulfilling my vocation in helping all these people.

Early glimmers of disillusion

But, little by little, a number of patients I thought I had cured returned three, four, or even five times over the course of a winter with the same condition. Colleagues practicing in the neighborhood told the same story. patients relapsed as soon as they stopped taking the medicine, which had prescribed according to the rules ordained by medical science. They presented with more not fewer complaints and developed other troubles they believed to come from their treatment. On examination, I heard the return of the wheezing, swollen tonsils once more, return of the stuffed-up nose, recurrence of pain, reappearance of eczema. The same patients occupying the same seats in the waiting room yet again.

I am appalled to see that today, 40 years later, every day in our country, the same patients continue to return to their physicians with the same complaints and relapses and suffer the same side effects.

After working for a few months, I started to experience a sense of futility about the kind of medicine I was practicing. I found myself disconcerted by the quizzical look in the eyes of my patients, as they asked:

- "Doctor, I don't understand why I am always ill …"
- "Doctor, you gave our baby antibiotics four times in a couple of months and he's still no better, and now they don't want him anymore at his crèche …"
- "Doctor, my headaches haven't got any better …"
- "Doctor, I feel even worse with your treatment …"

This couldn't go on any longer, I had to find a solution, both for them and for me.

Questions, but no answers

Like any doctor practicing medicine in an urban setting, I quickly had to come to terms with the reality of daily practice, with the disparity between the constant pressure of 30 to 40 patients a day, or even more, and the fine theoretical lectures I attended in medical school.

I soon came to realize that, in order to be time-efficient, "Doctor, there are still ten others in the waiting room," we doctors are conditioned to act mechanically like some kind of sorting machine: sick/ not sick, serious/not serious, urgent/not urgent. We "get a feel" for the patient more than properly examining them and often judge, simply from an intonation in their voice, whether or not it is an emergency. Otherwise, it is a well-rehearsed affair: renew the monthly prescription, hastily rewritten to "cover" the patient for hypothetical complications.

Soon, talking these things over with colleagues about the direction our practice was taking, I started to worry about prescription abuse, with long-term remedies casting their net too wide with the "same treatment" been given for the "same disease," as if each patient was "the same."

I began to ask myself about the sense of the rules imposed upon doctors which focus upon the disease being diagnosed rather than the person being treated. The implementation of such criteria, which completely remove the uniqueness of each individual from the equation, is monitored by officials whose job it is to verify that for such and such a disease the correct medicament has been prescribed, in accordance with the rulebook. As a consequence, physicians gradually lose the capacity to think for themselves. Their pen fills out the prescription unthinkingly, since the decision has already been taken beforehand, according to best practice guidelines (*Références médicales opposables*),[1] and consensus conferences.[2] It is not about the patient as a real person made of flesh and bone, it is only the disease they have that counts, and the financial cost. Economies must be made whatever the cost, because the healthcare budget is bursting at the seams. too bad if it is the patient who has to pay!

Long before today's pharmaceutical scandals (the withdrawal of drugs shown to be dangerous, doubts and being suspicions cast on others) I was looking for an alternative to the heedless prescription of powerful synthetic products. These, I thought, should be reserved for perhaps 10% of patients, who had genuine need of them. I pondered the possible consequences in the long-term of the overuse of such powerful pharmacological agents on such a large scale for such a huge number of patients. By blocking a function, or substituting for another with these drugs, we cannot know what their long-term disturbance on the regulatory systems of repair and defense in the human body. Could there be a less toxic therapeutic alternative better adapted to human needs? Is the medical system there to serve the patient, or the pharmaceutical companies?

So many answered questions led me to spend more time with each of my patients. I sensed that in order to do justice to every case and offer better treatment, I first had to develop an all-inclusive and personalized approach to their case. After less than a year of medical practice, I had had quite enough of treating them as ciphers and prescribing standardized treatments, ordered from on high.

And it was by talking to them and listening carefully to what they had to say, by seeing them as a whole person rather than focusing exclusively on the symptom that motivated their visit, I started to realize, little by little, that it is possible to practice another type of medicine. I developed a new outlook. It became clear to me that a hidden reality lay beyond the symptoms from which they suffered. Complex mechanisms had to be identified to fully understand the inherent strengths and weaknesses of their bodies so that the source of the imbalances which manifested in their troubles could be identified.

I also understood that I had to stop treating them like children. It was time to help them assume responsibility for maintaining their own health.

Encounters that would make all the difference

The scruples of a young general practitioner may seem derisory compared with the scale of the anticipated benefits promised by the great medical advances of the time, a period when fundamental research revealed some astonishing discoveries.

Let's not forget that the 1970s were a time of important breakthroughs.

- 1965: Jacques Monod, François Jacob, and André Lwoff were awarded the Nobel Prize for Medicine for their work on genetics and molecular biology, opening the way for research that would eventually lead to the deciphering of the human genetic code.
- 1966: the combined contraceptive pill became available in France.
- 1967: the first beta blockers were licensed for sale.
- 1967: the first heart transplant was performed by Christian Barnard in Cape Town, followed a year later by Professor Cabrol in France.
- 1972: a major new antibiotic, amoxicillin, was launched.
- 1974: Cefadroxil, another revolutionary anti-infective molecule, was first in use.
- 1976: the first MRI scanners: Magnetic Resonance Imaging revolutionized radiography, providing 2D or 3D imaging of the body.
- 1978: first "test tube baby" born by in vitro fertilization (IVF).
- 1980: Interferon, the first therapy using recombinant technology in production.

In short, huge technological advances in a little more than a decade, but they did little to resolve the doubts I had when facing the daily reality of my patients.

Then, as fate would have it, three doctors crossed my path who were destined to play a very important role in my life. The year 1972 had just begun. The recent student "revolution" of May, 1968, had ushered in a radical cultural, social and politic reappraisal of the traditional mores of our society, and that process was continuing apace. Ecological and environmental concerns fueled criticisms of the many negative aspects of modern life and stimulated a trend towards healthier living and a yearning for a return to nature. It was an era when new ideas proliferated.

In those heady days, one of my friends, a physiotherapist who treated the celebrities of the day, threw a little party for me which turned out to be a turning point in my medical evolution. He was well aware of my professional misgivings.

"I am going to introduce you to two doctors who furthermore are surgeons ... they are very remarkable, as you will see; I won't say more about them, but I've known them for a long time and I think you should meet them ..."

So it was that on one evening in February, 1972, I found myself in the company of these two individuals in the rooms of the Automobile Club in *Place de la Concorde*. Straightaway, these two doyens of surgery launched into a lively discussion.

The first, Jean Valnet, an enthusiastic and persuasive person, was very well known at the time for his books on herbal medicine. He had had an interesting career: during the war in Indochina, in the early 1950s, he had been an army surgeon at a French military hospital in Tonkin where he performed emergency operations on the battlefield. When he got back to Paris, he was appointed Chief Medical Officer to the Army General Staff and to the Cabinet of the Minister of the Armed Forces until 1959, when he decided to devote himself to the use of medicinal plants in private practice.

The second was Jacques Reynier. He had graduated as a brilliant young surgeon from the Paris Medical Schools, and then went on to make his name in the fields of breast and thyroid cancers and who, in a very few years, would become Head of General Surgery and Oncology at the Boucicaut Hospital.

I would never have imagined in a million years that one day he would call me to work alongside him for 7 years until his retirement. I could always count on his support and encouragement. he wrote the foreword to most of the books aimed primarily at the medical community that I have written in collaboration with colleagues, and towards the end of his career, he wanted me to join the Oncology Department of the Georges Pompidou European Hospital to continue the work he had inaugurated with us at Boucicaut.

The conversation between these two brilliant men soon became a battle of words. Valnet, who had practiced Phytotherapy in Paris for several years, made the spirited assertion that in the fullness of time, medicine would of necessity have to embrace medicinal plants. Reynier replied: "Sure, but look at the extraordinary progress that science is making: without the new antibiotics we wouldn't be able to operate on our patients. Modern surgery is unthinkable without these drugs."

Unperturbed, Valnet tried to outbid him: "you know, Jacques, when I was on the battlefield, I had injured people in a very bad way on the operating table, and something really puzzled me: how come that some of them developed no infection, and others, with the same kind of injuries, developed gangrene and needed amputation? I made inquiries, and the answer was always the same: those who had not succumbed to infection were those who had been treated by Vietnamese peasants with medicinal herbs, whereas the others had not. This was one of the reasons why, when I later joined the War Department, I began to pursue my interest in medicinal plants and started to use them to treat servicemen and their families."

Seeing my astonishment, he addressed me with military bluntness: "you're too young in this business (he was 22 years older than me) to understand this. You still believe in the omnipotence of science. But I have seen more sick people than you can imagine, and on whom the plants had such a positive effect that, even now, I cannot understand how it is possible. But it is true. For example, you can cure recalcitrant cystitis, which makes a misery of some women's lives, especially when antibiotics don't work, by giving the patient preparations of essential oil of lavender. They are often cleared of infection for good."

Both Jacques Reynier and I were taken aback by what he was saying. How was it possible for a surgeon, who seemed to have the head on his shoulders, to assert with such conviction that he can get rid of bacteria in urine by giving the patient perfume to drink!? But who were we to doubt the word of Valnet who, as he told us during our discussion, had recently been asked to treat Robert Boulin, the Minister of Health at the time?

The first glimmer of success

That meeting was the turning point of my professional life and marks the moment when, at last, I began to find some answers to my many questions, though the perspective was somewhat disconcerting to my scientific training: plants being sometimes more effective than antibiotics?! It took me some time to appreciate the prospects for better health that medicinal plants can offer when used wisely and supported by a reliable diagnosis. But during that meeting, my mind was in a whirl, for, during the course of the meal, Valnet suggested that I substantiate the truth of his empirical observations for myself and challenged me to take on a few patients and to see for myself.

So it was that a month later, the first of the patients sent by Jean Valnet came into my consulting room. She was a 40-year-old woman who had suffered from severe chronic cystitis since her teens. She had been seen for months by a urologist who had prescribed a course of long-term antibiotics, without any improvement. The bacteria clung resolutely to her bladder! I prescribed for her the simple magic formula that Valnet had jotted down on a piece of paper during our meal: tincture of bilberry and walnut with essential oils of lavender and juniper. That was all there was to it.

To my great amazement she returned for a follow-up consultation two months later and told me that ever since she had started on my plant-based prescription, all her symptoms had cleared up and no bacteria were detectable in her urine.

How could this be possible? In 1972, there were to my knowledge no scientific papers nor published reports that demonstrated the efficacy of medicinal plants against infection, and still less that they were more effective than antibiotics in treating a chronically sick person! Yet the laboratory test results were plain to see: for the first time in many years her urine had been free from bacteria.

These findings unnerved me, and I found it all very difficult to take in. I couldn't see how such a treatment could be so effective and wondered why my professors at medical school had never mentioned such alternative treatments? Perhaps they were not even aware of such phenomena; at that time, doctors didn't treat their patients with medicinal plants. the last 15 years had heralded an era in which chemistry triumphed, so plants were the last thing on the mind of medical scientists. The future lay with synthetic medicinal drugs.

Little by little, as I continued in practice, I began to grasp the huge potential that treatment with medicinal plants could offer me and my patients. But at the same time the truth began to dawn on me that things weren't quite that simple, and successful outcomes were less reliable than I had come to expect. Not all patients, by any means, showed a positive response to the plant-based formulas that Valnet detailed in his books. I soon began to see the limitations and drawbacks of this piecemeal kind of medicine that focused exclusively on symptoms. It had much in common with the formulations that naturopathic physicians publish in the mainstream press that are generic for this or that pain or complaint. The time had come for a critical analysis and to come to some understanding of the reasons for the success' as much as the failures. This was to be a long journey.

I spent many nights reflecting on how to make the transition between the "scientific" medicine I had been taught and "empiric" therapy based only on observation and my own personal experience, but which seemed to work, judging by the results obtained on a daily basis. There was also the fear of failure, and the responsibility to my patients.

The medicinal use of plants did not feature at all during our medical studies except to briefly mention that they had been abandoned because their effects were difficult to reproduce, and so, we were taught, their only benefit is to provide research chemists with molecules to work with. I spent my time reading and researching and my eyes were opened to the fascinating world of plants and the immense possibilities they offered us and which would come to dominate the next 40 years of my professional life. It took me years to come to grips with the complex actions that plants can exert on living organisms. I came to appreciate that to benefit fully from their potential, they need to be chosen only after deep reflection on the individual case, and then prescribed for their power to correct the imbalances in the terrain that was the root cause of the patient's disorder.

The third crucial encounter was with Christian Duraffourd, a young doctor like me who was also starting out in practice in Paris. His father, Paul Duraffourd, was a friend of Doctor Valnet. A biologist and pharmacist, he was Director of the Laboratory in the Department of Clinical Cardiology at Broussais Hospital.

Valnet, recognizing the benefit of having alongside him two young general practitioners who had already built up a good practice, introduced me to Christian Duraffourd in April, 1972. We both joined his newly-fledged Association of Phytotherapy, which he had set up following the great success of his book *Doctor Nature*.[3]

This was the beginning of a friendship and professional relationship that would last over 35 years. Our long and fruitful collaboration led us to create the concept of "Clinical Phytotherapy," which will be discussed in detail later. Clinical Phytotherapy is a new and original approach to the use of the medicinal plants that we developed in Europe and in other countries of the world. We decided to reconsider the use of medicinal plants without limiting them to addressing symptoms—one symptom, one plant—as is conventionally practiced by adepts of naturopathy without medical training (such as Rika Zaraï and others). It was this limited and simplistic view of plants that led to the abandonment of Phytotherapy by science-based medicine.

We were convinced that the use of medicinal plants would not achieve its full potential unless it were integrated into a global and comprehensive approach towards the human body and its physiology; this is why we coined the term "Clinical Phytotherapy."[4] Credibility for the therapeutic use of medicinal plants can be attained only within a scientific framework, such as the one that our training as general practitioners had provided.

A new concept

My collaboration with Christian Duraffourd was, from the very beginning, founded on our mutual approach to the treatment of the sick. By viewing each person in their totality, we shared a desire to develop what would become a true terrain-based medicine.[5]

I well remember Christian Duraffourd pondering on the notion of the patient's globality in his first year in practice. "You know, Jean-Claude, what really shocked me during my hospital internships was that at no time did my Department heads make the connection between the various systems maintaining equilibrium in the human body. In the morning, we were reminded how very complex, subtle, and finely-tuned the endocrine system was, and how we had to act with caution in view of this constant flux. But by the afternoon, it was as if they had forgotten everything! When they saw patients with a minor thyroid problem in their private practice, they would prescribe the same dose of levothyroxine as they had in the hospital.[6] They took no account of their individuality nor the eventual consequences that such doses could have on the rest of their bodies."

Some 30 years later, medical science has started to question the advisability of administering this medicinal product in the long-term with concerns about as yet unidentified secondary effects. In common with many other doctors, we observed the adverse reactions caused by this product as we followed patients over the years. It had been hurriedly prescribed for the tiniest nodule on the thyroid gland without due thought for the behavioral changes it might induce in women such as depression, weight gain, allergies, and menstrual disorders. It seemed very clear to us that this hormonal action on the thyroid as well as all the other endocrine glands would have to be damaging with long-term consequences that could not be ignored. But it took a long time for the regulatory authorities to recognize and accept this reality, which has contributed to the loss of trust from the public. Since January 31, 2011, AFSSAPS[7] has included levothyroxine on the list of medicinal products placed under "strict" control.

The delay in recognizing the adverse effects of this product, as with many others, comes from adopting a fragmented approach to the human body and therapeutic strategies that are non-integrative and which do not place a person's symptoms within the context of their whole lives.

We recognized this danger from the early days of practice. That is why we have oriented our research and practice towards a terrain-based medicine that would give a broader insight into the suffering person. An orientation that considers the patient in all their biological and human complexity, helping us find the specific imbalances that are the root causes of their disease. Ours is a theory of terrain in the true sense of the term and one which has clearly defined parameters, and so cannot be reduced to some fuzzy metaphor to cloak ignorance in the face of baffling illnesses. It is a terrain-based medicine that corresponds to a verifiable reality that can fully meet the requirements of modern science.

Our ideas grow and expand

Our practices were enriched by this new terrain-based medical approach and, in the course of time, our ideas were confirmed by clinical observation. We were encouraged to prepare the foundations for our first foray into imparting what we had learned. Doctors who had asked themselves similar questions to those that motivated us, were attracted by our approach and eagerly joined us. From 1980 we were all in agreement to focus our efforts on clinical and biological research into the mechanisms at play in the human body, and thereby construct a more comprehensive approach.

You cannot gain a deeper understand about the reasons for a loss of health without holding the complexity of the human being rigorously in mind. additionally, an approach intended to be comprehensive cannot afford to exclude any detail when searching out the reasons for the appearance of illness.

With this in mind we applied ourselves very early on to the study of external aggressors, whatever their nature: diet, hygiene and lifestyle, working conditions, daily and seasonal rhythms, toxins such as alcohol and tobacco, pollution from the air, as well as from chemical preservatives and other products, including medicines. We also considered the role of emotional aggressors, which have a considerable impact on the human body. Above all, we evaluated the role that endogenous aggressors had played in each individual case which had largely been ignored by modern medicine: the pathogenicity of their terrain, that is to say, their predisposition to develop such or such disease.[8]

Our second line of thought asked what approach should we adopt towards establishing a mode of treatment. We had to reconsider more deeply role natural products, medicinal plants in particular, could play alongside modern therapies and synthetic pharmaceutical medicines.

This was to be a long journey, with numerous pitfalls. together with the general practitioners trained in our vison of the integrity of the patient experience and in the properties of medicinal plants, we spent years in deliberation and verification. We had to validate our theories through the clinical observation of our patients and those of the practitioners in training. There were also confrontations, often animated, with our colleagues in French hospitals who sometimes called into question the direction our methodology was taking and where it might lead.

In 1985, at the request of the Ministry of Health and Social Affairs, we drafted a report on the state of the Phytotherapy in France. We also sat on many ministerial committees[9] with the remit of making a clinical assessment of the therapeutic benefits of medicinal plants, and to the feasibility of training general practitioners in their use. Throughout the 1980s we applied ourselves to communicate with the political, administrative, medical and professional authorities of our country. We also dedicated ourselves to teaching physicians. As well as in France, we organized private courses in England, Belgium, Italy, Mexico and the United States. We were also able to institute university courses in France at the University of Lille, in Greece in the Pharmacology Department of the Medical School in Athens, and in Tunisia at the School of Pharmacy in Monastir.

The launch of international congresses, such as the one we set up in collaboration with Professor Rachid Chemli in Tunis in 1993, allowed us to reach a larger audience and to lay the foundations for scientific partnerships with our Tunisian and Mexican friends. with 500 delegates from 49 countries—doctors, pharmacists, researchers, members of international and industrial organizations—after an overview of how medicinal plants are utilized around the world, we debated their future and their place in our healthcare systems, together with the scientific monitoring of their use.

An experiment in the treatment of cancer in a Paris Hospital

In 1989, many years after I had first met him, we got a telephone call from Professor Jacques Reynier. who by then had been appointed Chief of Staff at Boucicaut Hospital in Paris. He told us, "Listen guys, I've been following your progress for over 10 years. You send me a lot of cancer patients who need surgery. There are two types of cancer patients: those who obviously have cancer, and those who look fine and don't seem sick at all. When I open the door of the waiting room at my hospital, I can spot them right away. It turns out that the patients who do not seem to be ill are invariably patients in your care. So, I want to make you a proposition: I would like to offer you the opportunity to come and work with me in my Department. I am certainly not asking you to treat cancer with plants and oligo-elements, but I do want you to help my patients to tolerate chemotherapy better, and to recover more quickly from surgery."

Our attendance at Boucicaut would last for 7 years, during which time we treated a lot of patients. Professor Reynier managed to get the Paris Public Hospital System to officially appoint us as Research Associates of the *Assistance publique* and pay us each 150 Francs a month,[10] regardless of the time spent in his Department.

We didn't care about the money; we were fired up and ready to go. At last, other doctors would be able to judge for themselves the effectiveness of therapy with medicinal plants when founded on a personalized and comprehensive diagnosis of patients with very advanced disease. We were able to attend weekly meetings with surgeons, oncologists, radiotherapists, endocrinologists and other specialists. We learned a great deal, and new ideas were fermented, and we came up with some new approaches, all to further the greater wellbeing of patients.

After our first 2 years in the Department, we suggested that we publish a report to provide our explanation for the improvements experienced by many patients (according to the testimony of nurses and caregivers), following our supportive treatments. So, we produced a bimonthly booklet of some 30 pages that was circulated to surgeons and oncologists in which we explained in scientific terms the theoretical basis for treating each patient uniquely, and to elucidate the modalities of our approach, for which Professor Reynier coined the term "Oncobiology."

Some read it with curiosity and interest, other with skepticism, even dismissing the ideas out of hand. At that time, the medical community was still a long way from accepting ideas that are currently gaining positive attention: how natural therapies may benefit patients undergoing chemotherapy, and the importance of healthy lifestyle for cancer patients.

One of our colleagues, a young oncologist, was a proponent of aggressive chemotherapy. He was particularly hostile to the idea that a comprehensive approach to the terrain may give us a better understanding of cancer and still less that medicinal plants may could offer any benefit to patients. He was very angry when we gave him a copy of our publication *Oncobiology Factsheets*. In front of everyone, and in the presence of the Head of the Department, he dealt us the following blow: "What you are doing here in an Oncology Department with your terrain-based approach and your plants is completely unacceptable. As for your writings, see what I do with them ..." and, with a violent gesture, he threw the publication into the dustbin for all to see.

Times have changed since this episode. We are pleased to see that this colleague is now close to accepting our ideas that he once so vehemently rejected. He has recently taken up the cause of endocrine disruptors[11] and leads an aggressive campaign against pollutants and chemicals. We explained to him at the time the huge impact these substances could have on the terrain and the endocrine system and increasing the likelihood of cancer. He is currently head of a European cancer association, and we would be happy to see him taking a further step in our direction.

The 7 years spent in this Surgery and Oncology Department gave us much food for thought on so many questions. The most pressing issue was how to formulate objective measurements of the efficacy of our treatments based on global herbal extracts, which Professor Reynier had asked us to prepare to support his patients in their fight against cancer.

*Our search for the specific biological tool for assessing
the condition of the patient's terrain*

Colleagues and nurses at the Boucicaut Hospital had the distinct impression that patients were generally doing better since we had joined the Department. Patients coped better with chemotherapy, had fewer side effects and were less tired. But the claims for these improvements could not be established on opinions alone, however favorable they might be. To produce hard evidence, we would need to have at our disposal a biological tool of sufficient power and sensitivity to quantify the slightest physiological changes. Such a tool would help us diagnose the patient's condition very precisely in the first place and so offer some objective validation of our overall management of each case.

Secondly, it would need to validate—or fail to validate—by a methodology that was fully quantifiable that the biological changes attributable to our complementary treatments had actually taken place and were in accord with our clinical findings during our follow-up of patients. By way of an example, let's consider a less complicated condition than cancer, such as an allergic terrain, or tendency. Let's say that we a treat a patient for allergic rhinitis and on follow-up he seems to be cured of his runny or stuffed-up nose. In such a case, we would want to have a biological modeling tool that could demonstrate a diminishment of *total* histamine activity throughout the body in parallel with the clinical improvement. This would demonstrate a truly system-wide resolution and not just a suppression of local symptoms. We wanted to avoid the censure that any form of intuitive medicine might justify but rather build on firm foundations, verifiable within the hospital context.

It took the genius of Christian Duraffourd to devise a system that was capable of making a quantitative assessment of the patient's structural and functional state. The system provides a detailed mapping of the balances and imbalances at work in the body and generates a series of complex interrelated indexes. This elaborate scheme, which he christened the *Biology of Functions*, is based entirely on modern physiology and biology, as we shall see in Chapter 3.

New perspectives for patients and their doctors

A key feature of our professional lives was our wish to bring the results of our work, both in the hospital and in our private practice, to the attention of the medical and administrative authorities. We thought it most importance for our patients for us to make every effort to avoid provoking censure from the public health authorities.

Early in 2003, we met with the Dean of one of the Medical Schools in Paris, who had been charged with reform of medical training nationally. We presented him with a dossier in which we summarized the principal reasons we thought would justify the inclusion of the basic principles of Clinical Phytotherapy onto the medical curriculum. Few medical students would ever hear—unless as a joke—the words "medicinal plant" and fewer still would be exposed to the vaguest information about plants, the compounds they contain and their pharmacological action on the body, which is, after all, the basis of any medicament. Yet, as soon as they started in practice, they would be confronted with patients who, responding to media pressure that promoted a "return to nature," were very interested in so-called natural products, and medicinal plants in particular. Therefore, we thought it appropriate to offer at least a modicum of training on this subject so as to be able to provide an informed response to patients' questions on such matters.

In addition, we explained that in cases where it was appropriate to avoid powerful drugs, "Clinical Phytotherapy" and its use of medicinal plants can provide an effective alternative, but only after the necessary training. As we had over 10 years of teaching experience in Tunisia at the Faculty of Monastir, we offered to make our team of teachers available to the Department and begin the training in the next academic year, under the direct supervision of the appropriate medical and academic authorities. Eight years on, we are still waiting for a reply to our proposal.

Meanwhile, we have put all our effort into clinical work and to offering courses and seminars to spread the word on terrain-based medicine and Clinical Phytotherapy. As international exchange is an important instrument for developing multidisciplinary research, I continued to broaden my contacts abroad to compare our own results with those obtained by American, British, Mexican and Tunisian researchers or doctors who are applying the principles of our new medical approach in their practices.

To this end, besides establishing clinical training, I developed an expert system in close collaboration with my friend Patrice Pauly, that as well as allowing access to the Biology of Functions, provided a helpful tool to help apply it in everyday medical practice. This system is currently in use in the United States and Mexico by various teams of physicians involved in oncology, pediatrics, cardiology, and metabolic pathology.[12] It has been developed and expanded by data provided by over 30,000 biological tests done over the past 20 years.

While these results are receiving increased attention abroad, we cannot help wondering why France would brush aside methods that might bring hope to those that need it. For the wellbeing of patients, we want to make this new terrain-based approach available to the French doctors, and so offer them access to a system of personalized medicine, which has the additional merit of playing an important preventative role, as will be seen later in this book.

Prevention is a real issue, from the economic as much as the medical standpoint, given the growing deficit in Health and Social Security, made worse by the burden of serious disease.

It is time to have an open debate within our profession, and particularly with the decision makers. In this country where new ideas seem to meet with more resistance than elsewhere, one way forward is through a book like this, which is addressed in all sincerity to both patients and doctors alike.

CHAPTER TWO

Is evidence-based medicine supported by evidence?

From the origins of humanity to genetics

Since the beginning of humanity, we have taken our health and our life for granted. When disease strikes us, we are besieged by contradictory feelings: fear, trust, hope, resignation, and despair. Often guilt takes hold of us: *what have I done to deserve such a punishment?* This anguish could lead a person to think that the malign state taking hold of their bodies could be of supernatural origin.

In ancient times, invocation, prayer, and sacrifice were the first remedies. Distraught and powerless, the sick would appeal to a mediator who knew magic formulas and plants likely to ward off evil: the shaman. Rite, magic, sacrifice, and religion were conflated with medicine.

This intertwining of medicine and faith, with the priest as intermediary healer between those who suffered and supernatural forces, would gradually unravel over time. Faith and science progressively distanced themselves from one another and the supposed evil, stripped of its supernatural origin, was regarded as an exclusively natural phenomenon to be dealt with by rational means and advances in technology. Over the course of centuries, perceptions of health changed from symbolic and religious ones to a scientific approach. The European renaissance opened a new era that would last up to the end of the eighteenth century. Previously, man knew very little about his own body. The prohibition against the dissection of corpses, in force both in Christian and Muslim countries, rendered anatomical research impossible.

It was not until the sixteenth century, thanks to the work of Vesalius (1514–1564), considered as one of the pioneers of modern medicine, that the essential features of the macroscopic structure of the human body became accurately known. The invention of the microscope in the seventeenth century by van Leeuwenhoek (1632–1723), allowed the histological aspects of microstructures that had been observed by anatomists to be explored in much greater depth. The tremendous development of anatomy and surgery together with new analytical methods soon lead to the early major discoveries in physiology.

As we moved in the direction of analytical medicine with its success' and obvious benefits, less and less interest was shown in the globality of the human body. Thus, the vision of the body as a whole in balance with itself and in its relationship with its environment, an idea that had prevailed since the dawn of humanity, was abandoned.

This more holistic stance has been discredited and abandoned by modern medicine. The so-called "terrain-based" approach, often, it must be said, muddled and poorly understood, was regarded as a relic of an empirical past and had no practical importance and so was left in the hands of the back-to-nature movement, itself a response to the over reliance on machines and technology in modern medicine.

The concept of terrain or constitution

Yet the idea that each individual has a particular disposition to health and that illness takes a different form from one person to another has always existed. People may say: "he went down with pneumonia because of his constitution," or "his disease erupted suddenly out of the blue, but he got better quickly because he has a solid constitution," or on the contrary "he went quickly, because he had a weak constitution."

Medicine has been imbued with this notion of constitutional terrain since its origins. The absence of a clear definition of this nebulous and often misused term is the source of much confusion. You hear talk of terrain: the homeopathic terrain, the genetic terrain, the notion of terrain in Chinese, Tibetan, and Ayurvedic medicine, and so on, but what is the reality behind this concept that remains elusive both for the public and for doctors?

Hippocrates, who is regarded as the father of medicine, explained this predisposition to develop certain diseases by the existence of constitutions or idiosyncrasies. He defines health as the result of the balance between "bodily humors," a term which classifies all the fluids circulating in the body. These "humors" are four in number: blood, phlegm or lymph, yellow bile and black bile. According to the predominance of one or another of these humors, he established the existence of constitutions or temperamental types that gives each individual a certain physical conformation and tends towards a particular way of being: the four humors listed above are represented by the following types respectively: sanguine, phlegmatic, choleric and melancholic. The diseases people get, and the way they manifest, the intensity and course they follow are the consequences of how each temperament responds to aggressors and challenges.

The entire history of medicine developed around the notion that the constitution of the individual played an important role in the way he or she fell ill or, conversely, remained healthy when faced with aggressors.

In the nineteenth century, the work of Claude Bernard (1813–1878), founder of experimental medicine, highlighted the existence of the "interior milieu," an ocean of diverse liquids such as blood, lymph and cerebrospinal fluid in which the cells of the organism are bathed. This is the key to understanding "homeostasis," meaning that the internal conditions remain stable and balanced thus ensuring the maintenance of life. Disease occurs when this balance is compromised. In some ways, because of this idea of "internal sea," the Hippocratic theory of terrain seemed to be placed upon a more scientific basis.

Until the advent of the microscope in the Netherlands (Antoni van Leeuwenhoek 1632–1723) and England (Robert Hooke 1635–1703) the existence of microbes was unsuspected. It would still take a long time for the notion that disease was the result of a malfunction in the bodily humors to be replaced by the germ theory of disease. This was first proposed in 1840 by Friedrich Jakob Henle (whose influence on histology is comparable with that of Vesalius in anatomy). Three years earlier, Theodore Schwann had described the role of microbes in putrefaction and fermentation. Ten years later, Ignaz Semmelweis inaugurated the practice of antiseptic obstetrics in Hungary and saved many lives (though sadly not his own).

It was Louis Pasteur (1822–1895) who fully confirmed the germ theory of disease and was responsible for its wide dissemination.

Joseph Lister, who pioneered aseptic surgery, took his inspiration from his French contemporary. Pasteur placed bacteriology on an institutional footing and revolutionized medicine by applying his own discoveries and those of Robert Koch to public health policies. His demonstration that microbes caused anthrax and other diseases like tuberculosis and cholera ushered in an era of intense research with the discovery of the causative organisms of infectious diseases, for example, *Pneumococcus* for pneumonia, *Meningococcus* for meningitis. This led in turn to the hunt for molecules that were capable of destroying them. First in their sights were the bacteria, yeasts and fungi, like *Escherichia coli*, *Proteus*, *Klebsiella*, *Candida albicans*, all of which had been identified under the microscope. Later, thanks to advances in biology and technology, came the viruses, which, being so much smaller were much more difficult to identify. Before long, the presence of a microorganism, isolated and precisely described in the laboratory, came to be associated with a particular disease: the germ becomes responsible for the disease and became identifiable with it. Thus, the so-called "specific etiology theory" was born, associating a precise, measurable, and unique cause with each disease.

The analytical approach very quickly found its way into all areas of medicine. For a metabolic disorder, one sought the defective enzyme, for hormonal abnormality, the dysregulated hormones, and for a congenital malformation: the faulty gene.

The advances in knowledge that accrued from the scientific method set the course for modern medicine to follow. It involved fragmenting the human body into its very smallest parts and focusing research on each functional mechanism. Thus, it led to reducing the living being into a simple sum of components isolated from their context, much easier to study than their complex functioning within the integrated system to which they belong, the human body as a whole.

From the complexity of the whole to the study
of its infinitely small components

This fragmented view of the human being led to segmenting the body into its constituent parts. This in turn led doctors to gradually turn aside from an overarching view as they moved away from looking at the entire human body and started to focus on organs, then the tissues that formed those organs, then from there to the constituent cells.

But the cell itself is composed of a large number of smaller parts, from the mitochondrion and Golgi bodies to the nucleus and ribosome, all of them interacting via a multitude of ceaseless mechanisms and pathways. The need to go ever deeper into analyzing these microstructures tended to lose sight of the unity of the cell as a whole entity.

The cell is the building block of life. We had to invent new techniques, even new sciences in order to understand how billions of interactions can function in unison. These increasingly sophisticated methods gave birth to molecular biology and genetics. We have reached the ultimate limit of analysis as we have arrived at the fundamental molecules that constitute every component of living matter. Researchers have thus made of the cell a new Tower of Babel.

They have made a difficult challenge for themselves in that, they have lost sight of the unifying elements that integrate the parts to create a system. They have obscured the understanding of how the laws governing the genetic material at the smallest scale are reconciled with those governing whole-body systems in a coherent manner that facilitates the harmonious functioning of the whole living being.

This is one of the major problems created by modern medicine: by endlessly fragmenting the human body into its constituent parts and separating the part from the whole, it is unable to put all the pieces together again, to reconstruct the totality. Both the patient having to cope with the treatment and the doctor trying to understand the disease have been handicapped by this disastrous trend. The history of genetics illustrates this development very well.

Genetics: a triumph of technology more than a progress for patients?

I began my studies in medicine in 1961, at about the same time that Jacob, Monod, and Lwoff were working on the elucidation of the transcription of the genetic code for which they went on to share the Nobel Prize.[1] I remember having to answer a question in my first-year examination about the mechanism whereby DNA was transcribed by messenger RNA. Barely 15 years had elapsed since the double helix structure of DNA had been discovered by Crick and Watson. These were new discoveries, and I was fascinated by the elegance and intelligence of the human body, but I could have no idea of the huge distance that medical science would travel over the next 40 years.

At that time, we had some idea about how cells functioned. We knew it to be organized like a miniature factory, that it had specialized structures for the production, storage and transport of nutrients, and manage to manage the flow of energy so that life could be maintained. But new and more complex research would penetrate the subtle innermost workings of the cell, giving rise to disciplines that went even further: Developmental Genetics, Quantitative Genetics, Population Genetics, Genomics, Proteomics, Transcriptomics, Metabolomics, the list goes on.

The ultimate goal was to decrypt the genome of each human being and understand how it operated so that the molecular defects that cause disease, from the relatively benign to cancer, could be discovered and corrected by genetic means. The complete sequencing of our genome would allow for the creation of new generation of innovative drugs, at least this is what scientists believed.

Science seemed to hold out the promise of before long finding the solution to all our ills. Thanks to the development of increasingly sophisticated techniques, one discovery followed another at a tremendous rate, and seemed to justify such hopes. However, as the research became more sophisticated and our detailed knowledge of our body at the microscopic scale deepened, we became less and less able to make any grand synthesis of the information so acquired, or to connect the parts and integrate them into a comprehensive vision of the human being. The genome is more complex than a simple user's manual. To quote Jim Collins, a biologist at the University of Boston, the head of the National Institutes of Health (NIH): "We made the mistake of confusing the collection of information with an improvement in our understanding."[2]

We need, therefore, to return to an older, more comprehensive approach. We believe the time has come for a move in the opposite direction; to start from the whole and try to understand, in an integrated way, how to transpose and construe the amazing discoveries made by analytical science. To do this, we must first be clear about the key data this scientific revolution has brought to our understanding of living beings.

A brief overview of genes

Genetic information in all living creatures is contained in the chromosomes, and these are situated within the heart of the nucleus of the cell. Each one of the trillions of cells in the human body contains the identical genetic information, half coming from the mother and the other half from the father. We have 46 chromosomes in each cell; together, they make up our genome, which determines all our visible and invisible characteristics. Each chromosome is made of a very long strand of DNA (Deoxyribonucleic acid): a thread which is almost 2 meters (6.56 feet) long, folded into the nucleus, a space only a few thousandths of a millimeter in diameter. Along these threads are written the many lines of code that contains our body plan by orchestrating the synthesis of enzymes that control each stage of every biochemical metabolic pathway, as well as the construction of our tissue proteins.

In the early days of nuclear microscopy, the nature of these irregularly bunched chromosomes (which means "colored bodies" because they were visualized by colored dyes) was not really understood. We now know that a single strand of the molecule, made up of a string (or polymer) of nucleic acids, takes the shape of a helix that is coupled with another complementary strand to make up a pair. The two strands are united into a kind of twisted ladder joined by "rungs" made of a sugar called deoxyribose together with a phosphate, which gives a certain rigidity to the molecule. The rungs of the ladder contain the genetic information, encoded in four distinct

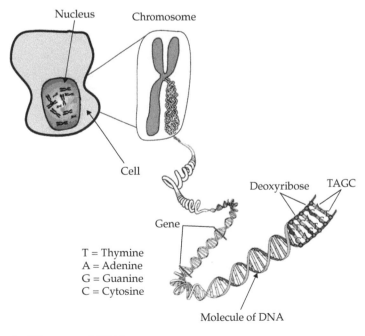

Figure 1: Diagram of DNA.

chemicals: Adenine (A), Thymine (T), Cytosine (C), and Guanine (G). These are technically nucleotides but are generally known as bases.

The "language" of DNA is a code that is written using just these four "letters," or, bases, which always associate in the same pairs, thus: Cytosine on one strand is always matched with a Guanine facing it on the other (C-G); likewise Thymine with Adenine (A-T).

The nucleus of each cell in our body contains a molecule of DNA, each double-strand having an estimated 3.5 billion pairs of bases. The sequence of the four "letters" can be arranged in a huge number of different ways and certain sections of this sequence constitute an instruction to the cellular machinery to synthesize a particular protein. Each separate instruction is called a "gene" and is a code or message that may be switched on or off by yet other genes. DNA is effectively a series of messages, which contain very accurate information that controls all the particular characteristics of our body, for example the color of the eyes, and does so by the ordered production of certain proteins. Human DNA contains approximately 20,000 different genes, each of them formulated by a sequence of just these four "letters." These genes are distributed across the DNA, and each has a precise and invariable physical location (or *locus*) on one of the chromosomes, and allows the genetic map of an individual to be assembled.

One would need thousands of pages to write a short novel if you only had four letters in your alphabet rather than the 26 letters we are used to. As the genetic alphabet does indeed contains only four letters, thousands of bases are needed to "write" the instruction represented by a single gene: cystic fibrosis spans approximately 230 kilobases (kb) (230,000 bases) and hemophilia 186 kilobases (186,000 bases). A genetic disease can be triggered by a single error in the sequence that constitutes the message for constructing an enzyme or structural protein.

The genes and our diseases: more questions than answers

Mutations or mistakes in the sequences that make up one section of the DNA molecule can occur at any time, in any cell in the body, either spontaneously during the copying process known as replication, or under the influence of some noxious agent, which may be chemical or physical. Examples of these so-called "mutagens" are damaging ultraviolet rays or tobacco smoke. When they affect only a small region of our chromosomes, we talk about genetic mutations; such mutations are modifying the sequences of the normal genetic program. The message the gene contains is then modified by these mutations and the effects may be quite slight. Some mutations, however, result in the production of damaged proteins, may be more significant and lead to illness of varying severity.

Fortunately, our body is able to repair the majority of these mutations, but sometimes they are not repaired and the mutated protein "binds" to the DNA and if this occurs in our reproductive cells, their effects can then be passed down to our offspring. However, if they appear in other types of cell, such as bone or liver, these anomalies will not be transmitted, but based on their severity, they may cause disease, for example cancer, in bones or liver.

There are other mutations whose effect on the genome is massive which can even alter the number or structure of chromosomes: for example, Down's syndrome is characterized by trisomy in chromosome 21, which means that there are three copies rather than the usual two. Then there are the so-called monogenic disorders, where a mutation in a single gene indicates a very high probability of triggering the disease occasioned by this error. Examples include Huntington's disease, cystic fibrosis, and certain diseases of muscle (known as myopathies). But not all subjects carrying this faulty gene will go on to develop the full-blown expression of the "same" disease. Each individual will develop the condition in their own way, with idiosyncratic signs and responsiveness to treatment.

This finding is very important because it shows that other factors are involved in modulating the expression of the pathological potential of this gene. This means that even in case of a highly penetrant gene—one that deeply affects how the body functions—the disease has other interactions than exclusively to the specific gene. This raises the question of the relationship with the external environment, and also with the overall physiological condition of the individual. It complicates infinitely the understanding of the relationship between the gene and the condition of the individual. Especially since we know that only a small part of our DNA (about 5%) corresponds to genes, and we do not know yet the function of the remaining 95%! In most cases, these mutations do not exhibit pathogenicity and do not have any detectable consequences. These are the so-called genetic polymorphisms, which play an important role, for example, in establishing paternity or in the use of genetic fingerprinting by forensic experts to identify a suspect. The victims of the terrorist attack on the World Trade Center in New York were identified using the so-called SNP (Single Nucleotide Polymorphism) detection techniques.[3]

The myth of "everything is genetic"

From the beginning of genetic research, the approach taken by Pasteur towards disease was considered by geneticists to be the most appropriate to medicine. They were convinced that the decryption of the genome would very quickly allow them to identify abnormal genes and thus to cure the patient by correcting the genes.

They were quickly disappointed; the reality did not match this simplistic approach. The complexity was soon revealed, thus upsetting the simplistic myth of "all genetics," which melted away like snow in summer. Little by little, the researchers discovered that even if the DNA is important as a carrier of genetic information, the adverse or neutral effect of a genetic mutation and its impact on the protein it encodes could only occur in a given environmental context. Such environmental context refers *mainly* to the overall internal physiological environment (terrain) of the individual carrier of the pathological gene, and secondarily to the external environment which makes demands on the internal one. The error, which prevailed for too long, was to believe *a priori* that everything was determined by the genes, and to consider that there is a direct cause-and-effect relationship between the presence of a specific gene and the existence of a certain disease.[4] Due to the complexity of all the phenomena at work within the human body, this reductionist view has been very seriously questioned.

Certainly, the so-called multifactorial disorders, such as cardiovascular disease and hypertension, obesity and diabetes, inflammatory disease and cancer, often involve the simultaneous presence of numerous genes. But each individual gene in isolation is neither necessary nor sufficient to cause the disease. This is amply shown by the fact that the same mutation may cause diseases of very different degrees of severity, or the same disease may be caused by anomalies in several genes. The disease seems to appear when a certain "threshold" of susceptibility is exceeded and is the result of the intricate action of genetic and environmental factors.

This explains why the illusion of the direct relationship between the presence of a specific gene and the so-called diseases of civilization had to be abandoned. Even so, hardly a day goes by without some sensational headline in the mainstream media: "Spectacular Breakthrough; The Connection Between Gene X With Disease Y Has Been Uncovered!," "New Gene Causes Prostate Cancer," "Hope in the Fight

Against Cholesterol: a New Gene Has Been Identified." Such "discoveries" arouse false hopes in the minds of their readers, convinced that some new "gene deletion therapy," soon to be available to all, will solve all their health problems.

Even if this "everything is down to genetics" notion had some predictive value, the assessment of risk and probabilities does little in itself to making medicine preventative. Even if being alerted to potential anomalies might offer some degree of prevention, a single observation cannot be enough on its own: it must be coupled with a genuinely preventative treatment.

And anyway, what does genetics really do for a patient, given the current state of knowledge? Genetic information provides a set of probabilities and not a specific diagnosis. If your tests show that you carry four abnormal genes, it means that you run some risk of developing four different diseases, then, it is a reasonable to pose the following question: is the geneticist able to prescribe you a preventative treatment that could correct each of the four detected anomalies? The truth is that medicine can offer no preventative treatment because it does not know the mechanisms that activate the genes. It can only detect. It cannot prevent the activation of the gene, much less cure the disease it is associated with. You are left alone with your risks and your fear of seeing these predictions materialized, perhaps tomorrow, perhaps never.

Diseases and genetic tests: prediction or probability?

As soon as geneticists discovered that the chromosomes were carriers of information, they tried to develop genetic tests to identify the specific characteristics of each individual. So-called "pre-symptomatic" tests are employed to determine if a person, apparently in good health, is or is not a carrier of genetic disease. "Susceptibility" tests assess the likelihood of the occurrence of a disease which may have multiple causes, but will often involve a genetic anomaly. Finally, "predisposition" tests are looking for the genes involved in the high-risk familial diseases; nevertheless, their presence does not mean that the disease will certainly develop.

Armed with these tests, geneticists hope to identify anomalies carried by the subject and develop treatments to correct them. A major goal hopes to develop so-called "predictive medicine," that will identify the genetic factors responsible, according to current thinking, for all conditions associated with all known diseases. But the reality is actually much more complicated because, as already mentioned, the genetic anomaly may be caused by several mechanisms, and there is no ready-made rule for predicting the severity of a mutation whatever its nature.

Genetic testing can assess the probability that a disease will occur but never with certainty: data provided by your genome can only evaluate your chances of developing certain diseases. Such a disease may befall you next month or in 20 years, or never, because nobody knows when.

Are genetic tests available on the internet a fraud?

It is very easy to find laboratories on the internet that provide a readout of your genetic blueprint and offer to quantify your predispositions and risks based on your genome, and to trace your genealogy and the geographical origin of your ancestors. To establish their credibility, they cite various scientific publications that document the fundamental research and present them as a guarantee of their validity. You send your saliva sample in a tube, along with your payment for analysis and maybe also an annual subscription to the service. The results are returned by mail, some six to eight weeks later:

Dear Ms. Smith

You are 20 years old; here are the results of the analysis of your genome. We have assessed your risks of expressing a hereditary or non-hereditary disease, and your sensitivity to certain drugs, and your tendency to certain behavioral traits ...

You are 1.98 times more likely than average to develop Alzheimer's disease, 1.37 times more likely compared to the average to develop multiple sclerosis, 1.25 times more likely to develop biliary cirrhosis, 1.23 times more likely to develop psoriasis, 1.22 times more likely to develop stomach cancer ...Your chance of developing glaucoma is 0.8 times the norm, rheumatoid arthritis 0.79 times the norm, type-1 diabetes 0.11 times the norm, Crohn's disease 0.1 times the norm, and so on.You do not carry the genes causing Fanconi Anemia, Tay Sachs disease, Gaucher disease, breast cancer (gene BRC1) ... the list continues.

Regarding your sensitivity to medicinal products, you may experience side effects after administration of metformin, nausea

and vomiting after surgery, an addiction to heroin, a strong reaction
to Flucloxacillin, etc.

You probably have blue eyes and are highly sensitive to alcohol.
You are highly responsive to the HIV virus but not, by contrast, to
hepatitis B. Your athletic performance is poor. You have a high risk
of an early menopause, a tendency to produce cerumen (earwax),
and, all things being equal, you can expect a long life …

Don't you think this information will give poor Ms. Smith reasons
enough to be concerned? What can she do with all this information and
set of probabilities? So, she may be 1.98 or 1.22 more likely to be the
victim of such and such a serious illness, perhaps by the age of 30, but,
of course, this is not certain as she may live to be 100! And what can
her doctor do with these figures for which no preventative treatments
exist for the potential disasters mentioned? It is worth pointing out that
this supposed science, occupying a somewhat "recreational" niche, has
moved the French Society of Human Genetics to publish a document
warning the consumer of the "scientific limitations or even the down-
right errors that may follow the inappropriate interpretation of such
test results, and the potential risks that may ensue."

The ethical pitfalls of genetic testing

The ethical dangers posed by the inappropriate use of genetic tests soon
came to light. Let's not forget the animated debate in the French Parlia-
ment in 2007 occasioned by the Mariani amendment to the immigration
bill, which sought to introduce DNA testing for all foreign applicants
seeking reunification with their families, a project that was fortunately
abandoned. A similar controversy occurred shortly afterwards in Great
Britain, over a project aimed at preventing fraudulent claims by asylum
seekers arriving from Kenya, by establishing their true nationality from
these same DNA tests. There are many other situations with potential
risks: the selection of candidates for a job, violation of an individual's
right to privacy by analyzing stolen hair, the setting of insurance premiums, and so on. To try to avoid such abuses, the rules stipulate that
"tests which are held to be predictive of genetic diseases, or which
serve either to identify the subject as a carrier of a gene responsible
for a disease or to detect a genetic predisposition or a susceptibility to
a disease can only be conducted for medical purposes or for medical
research, and must be made subject to appropriate genetic counseling."

In reality, things are not so straightforward, and the public faces a potential of discrimination when it comes to insurance premiums. The French Federation of Insurance Companies signed a 5-year moratorium obliging their members to refrain from resort using the genetic profiles of their customers when setting premiums. This moratorium was renewed in 1999. For the time being, insurance companies do not require genetic tests (except for Huntington's disease in some countries). On the other hand, they do require those seeking insurance cover to sign a declaration certifying that applicants are not suffering from any particular disease. There is no guarantee that this will continue in the future. Because of the steep rise in the rates of cancers and degenerative diseases, and the exponential rise in the costs of treating them, it quite possible that Life Insurance will only be made available to those with genes of low pathogenicity, while those with high-risk genes for diseases that are expensive to treat, will be declined cover.

Why are some people hypersensitive to certain medicinal compounds?

In 2007, a study conducted by the regional pharmacovigilance centers (EMIR[5]) in France revealed that the annual number of hospitalizations due to adverse effects of medicinal products amounted to 143,915, which represents an annual average of 1,480,885 days of hospitalization.

Given the scale of the problem, it is important to identify the reasons which could have led to such adverse reactions, and to find some way to eliminate them. We need to understand why the same medicinal product produces severe side effects in one patient, and not in another.

The answers to these inquiries will vary. The reactions may be age-related or due to the severity of the disease, to the kind of food in the diet, or an interaction with another drug being taken at the same time. It is also possible that the patient failed to take the correct dose, in which case the adverse effect is not surprising. However, quite often, patients who adhere to the correct dose scrupulously experience a wide range of disorders, of varying degrees of severity and duration, and go on to develop a permanent sensitivity to the product. What is the cause of such sensitivities?

It is well known that each of us has a different sensitivity to alcohol. One may be able to drink three glasses of whiskey without batting an eyelid and continue to drink while another is unsteady after one glass of champagne. This phenomenon is explained by the fact that the former is a "fast acetylator" with an inherited ability to rapidly break down and metabolize the alcohol, while the other is not. This is the reason why Asians and others who are "slow acetylators" have low tolerance to alcohol. We are not equal regarding alcohol and neither are we equal regarding medicinal products!

Pharmacogenetics suggests that differences in the genome play a major role in the way an individual processes and reacts to a medicinal compound. These constitutional differences between genomes may substantially influence a drug's efficacy and toxicity. The genetic tests being developed that are designed to find the tailor-made solution for an individual patient appear quite promising. However, as we have already noted, just as the correlation between the presence of an abnormal gene and the expression of a disease cannot be guaranteed, so there is no absolute correlation between the presence of a gene and the efficacy or toxicity of a certain medicinal product. The human body is very complex and has many compensatory strategies by which it can avert difficult situations, and genetic factors are by no means the only ones to influence our response to medicinal drugs which have complex actions on our bodies.

Any medicinal compound must first be absorbed for it to act, and then it has to be eliminated. We have special organs, the emunctories, charged with eliminating everything we ingest, whether food or medicament. The liver plays a crucial role here. this emunctory operates like a veritable factory with the responsibility for processing all the waste products of metabolism. However, three-quarters of all medicinal products are broken down by a group of enzymes, the so-called cytochrome P450 enzymes, found mainly in this organ, and genetic variations in an individual's genome may alter their action. This is why a patient who metabolizes the medicinal substance into a pharmacologically inactive substance more rapidly is much less likely to suffer serious side effects than one whose slower enzymes allow the toxic compound to build up in the body.

In oncology, this kind of research is particularly important as people who may already be very ill are exposed to very active molecules with powerful effects. In addition, anticancer protocols often combine two or three, or even four chemicals in a single chemotherapy session. This increases the risk of interactions not only between the chemotherapy agents themselves but also, in a more complex way, with the body's metabolic systems. Certainly, the genetic makeup of each subject will influence the response of each patient to the treatment, but we should not ignore the role of the functional state of the patient's organs and the general state of the body. This, as much as the genetic potential, has such an important effect on the activity of the enzymes that catalyze the biotransformation of these powerful drugs.

Establishing the genetic profile of an individual allows us to select the most suitable treatments for that patient's profile, and to avoid those that may be more harmful. Such genetic tests, known as DNA microarrays, already exist and are currently in use. For example, 18 variations of two genes that code for enzymes have been discovered. These are enzymes that metabolize the drugs involved in the metabolism of anti-hypertensive compounds as well as some antidepressants and anticonvulsants. But, as we have seen, genes are by no means the sole factors that dictate the course a disease will take or a patient's response to treatment: a comprehensive clinical approach to the follow-up of the patient is most important.

The reason for presenting this overview of genetics has been to show that an ultra-reductionist view of biology cannot envision the human body as a whole and, by focusing exclusively on genes has great difficulty in arriving at an understanding of how the body actually works and how it may fall from health and become ill.

Gene therapy: bubble babies success?

If the relationship between gene and disease is not as direct as once believed, the links between disease and gene therapy[6] are much more difficult to identify and the benefits, if any, are quite unpredictable.

During a Telethon in December, 1999, much publicity was given to the success of gene therapy developed by Professor Alain Fischer and conducted since 1993 at Necker Hospital to treat four "bubble babies." These are children born with severe immunodeficiency; their inability to make white blood cells obliged them to live in a totally sterile environment. Unfortunately, 2 years later, the treatment had to be halted because two of the treated children developed leukemia.

In May, 2004, because of the apparent promise of this therapeutic approach, AFSSAPS authorized the resumption of a modified protocol using improved retroviral vectors.[7] But complications reoccurred so the new therapy had also to be discontinued in 2005. As Professor Fischer's[8] statement is relevant: "It is absolutely clear that gene therapy is not *the* therapy. It is just an approach among many others … The basic principle is the evaluation of the risk to benefit ratio of our gene therapy compared with conventional therapy."

Although by April, 2010, no gene therapy product had received approval by the U.S. Food and Drug Administration (FDA), in June of the same year 1,644 clinical trials were conducted worldwide, 44 of them in France. Despite the absence of clear benefits, in 2015, the worldwide gene therapy market was estimated to be worth $500 million.

This is a strange success story when a therapeutic method that after 30 years of research, carried out around the world by thousands of researchers, has yet to provide clear evidence of any real therapeutic breakthroughs.

Given all this, we can only agree with Bertrand Jordan, founder of Génopole Marseille-Nice and a member of the European Molecular Biology Organization (EMBO[9]) when he wrote: "With all the media hype regarding stem cell therapy, and therapeutic cloning by nuclear transfer, one can only expect it to lead to profound disappointment."[10]

Evidence-based medicine and contemporary drug scandals

To understand the source of the failures in contemporary industrialized medicine we should see that they originate in an inability to make the transition from an analytical approach to a modality that creates a synthesis.

The expectation of the mechanistic methodology when treating ill people is for the body to return to its normal function by replacing damaged material with a spare part or by bearing down upon some biochemical mechanism that has wandered out of kilter, on the analogy to working on the engine of a car. But the human body does not work like a machine because in a living organism everything is interconnected and interdependent, so that when disease strikes, the "part" that seems to fail reflects a precarious state of the whole system. Artificially changing the part or blocking the mechanism will inevitably lead to a response of the whole body, which now must accommodate, or "digest" as it were, the aggression represented by the therapeutic act. The gene is not the equivalent of the disease, and even less with the patient as the carrier of that illness.

In most cases, therefore, single gene therapy is quite unsuitable as a treatment for sickness, except theoretically in exceptional situations where a structural monogenic disorder prevails. Conditions such as

Huntington's disease, colonic polyposis, or Marfan syndrome, are caused by a deficit in a single gene. Even if a specific gene therapy is developed for these rare diseases, that should not prevent us from also considering the totality of the individual.

By reducing the patient to a collection of parts, the analytical method is in danger of visualizing only the disease and forgetting that there is a person behind the disorder. The motive behind viewing conditions in the abstract, be they high cholesterol, cancer, diabetes, or rheumatism, lies in the hope of eradicating them. This unalloyed analytical method deliberately abandons all the specific characteristics of the individual, his or her medical history, previous illnesses, diet, idiosyncratic response to aggressors, lifestyle, social environment, work, and so on.

This simplistic view of the reality of the human being has also led to the emergence of so-called evidence-based medicine. Created by Anglo-Saxons, evidence-based medicine is defined as "the judicious use of current best evidence from clinical research to ensure personalized care of each patient."[11] Now, what qualifies as evidence?

The evidence is provided by systematic clinical studies, such as randomized controlled trials,[12] meta-analyzes, as well as cross-sectional studies or cohort studies (also known as Prospective Observational studies) or Case-control studies that are assumed to be reliable. And how are these studies and these protocols designed? They are based on the same analytical approach that focuses on the disease at the expense of the individual patient. It is a protocol-based medicine.

At first sight, this approach seems to have a lot going for it. First name the disease, then choose patients who all have this "same" disease, then test a product on them to see whether it will be effective or not. In a randomized placebo-controlled and double-blind study,[13] the results are then analyzed and the conclusions published. They might typically read, for example, that statistically, the medicinal product being tested is active in 45% of patients having the "same" disease.

Nevertheless, designing a study is not without problems. Allocating individuals to a group where the protocol dictates that they all have the "same" disease is, even by established inclusion criteria, utopian given the great diversity of human beings. Analyzing the effects of a treatment administered to hundreds of patients without considering their unique structural functionality, or the details of each individual diet, introduces considerable bias into the protocol, knowing full well that the interference of all these elements may change the metabolism of the compound to be tested, and thus its efficacy.

No patient is identical with another, and although they are said to carry the "same" disease, their reaction to what indeed is an identical molecule being tested may be very different because of the specificity of their condition. However, the activity of the remedy is evaluated only in relation to the disease. This explains why the occurrence of serious side effects is to be expected, since once the study has been completed, this molecule that has been tested on statistical criteria will be marketed along the same lines, and will be prescribed to all those who have the "same" disease. We may have to wait until it has been very widely distributed, which may take years, for these adverse, indeed highly toxic side effects to be officially recognized.

When one witnesses the disastrous side effects of some of our modern medicines, is it not reasonable to question the validity of randomization and double-blind techniques, which, we are told "have undeniably done much to ensure the rigor of studies and the safety of their therapeutic applications."

What are these guarantees of safety worth when drugs that make the headlines with a lot of razzmatazz have to be withdrawn from sale a few years after being given approval? We are told to begin with that the risk to benefit ratio of these new products is decidedly in favor of the benefits, and they are hailed as revolutionary medicinal products.

An example is provided by the story of the infamous Vioxx, which received its marketing authorization allowing it to be distributed in the European market in 1999. This was an anti-inflammatory medicine that, having successfully passed all the tests for efficacy and safety, was launched with massive publicity onto the market. It was championed as an example of the most sophisticated pharmacological and clinical research, and voted the MEDEC[14] "Medicine of the year" Prize for 2003 by over 6,000 French general practitioners.

Yet, as early as July, 2000, the French independent journal *Préscrire*, which does not receive any medical sponsorship, had warned consumers of its potential dangers. Despite further warnings issued after 2001, AFSSAPS (the French watchdog for Safety of Health Products) allowed this product to remain on the market. It took until September 30, 2004 for this showpiece of modern science to be withdrawn from international markets, after being officially recognized as responsible for over 140,000 cardiovascular events and 60,000 deaths in the United States, and 1,000 cases of adverse effects and the death of 32 patients in France. The Mediator® scandal,[15] in which the full extent of conflicts of interest within the pharmaceutical industry was to be exposed had not yet surfaced.

Celebrex, which contains a compound from the same family of cyclooxygenase-2 (COX-2) inhibitors as Vioxx®, and is indicated for "the symptoms of mild–to–moderate osteoarthritis," has curiously escaped the ban, although it produces serious side effects. These had already been reported several times in scientific journals and in the medical press. AFSSAPS' decision of 2011 to maintain this product on the market despite extensively documented side effects detailed in the Drug Information System (known as Vidal) may seem reckless in view of the cardiovascular risks in rheumatic patients. Given that these conditions are not life-threatening, is the recourse to such a powerful and potentially dangerous chemical treatment really justified? Especially when it is known that well designed plant-based therapies devoid of such dangers may provide an effective alternative. And what about the official list of 77 potentially dangerous medicinal products drawn up by AFSSAPS[16] that have been available on the internet since March, 2011?

Let's look at two anti-diabetic drugs, Actos® and Competact®, still prescribed in France to 230,000[17] patients annually. Writing in May, 2011 for *Figaro Madame*, the journalist Anne Jouan asked why AFSSAPS did not prohibit their use since the Pharmacovigilance Commission had recommended on March 29, 2011 that they be immediately withdrawn from the market given that they were at risk of inducing bladder cancer in addition to other known adverse effects, such as weight gain, congestive heart failure, edema and fractures. It was not until June 9, 2011 that these two medicines were withdrawn from the market.[18]

Isoméride®, Mediator®, Pondéral, and other weight loss drugs that had previously been praised to the skies were disowned by the medical world. The antidepressant Upstene®,[19] which had been awarded the Prix Galien for research in 1983, an award that celebrated "a distinguished tradition of excellence in pharmaceutical research," sank into oblivion as did other medicinal products that had been withdrawn because of their toxicity. The withdrawal of drugs for causing serious harm is not a new phenomenon, but new cases tend to highlight the risks of these medicines, despite all the precautions taken in their development.

It is as if a veil had been lifted on a health system that had been reassuring and beyond reproach, a smooth-running and well-ordered system. Who could have imagined the successive failures in the chain of accountability that starts off with the medicinal product being placed on the market and ends up with its prescription by the physician, in whom the patient has placed their trust?

Who could have thought it possible, without being taken for a conspiracy theorist, that experts could be both judge and in the dock, because while in the pay of pharmaceutical laboratories, they may take the decision to curtail clinical trials, to produce sham results, and co-opt poorly informed doctors?

But the real problem is not so much restricted to conflicts of interest and the covert malpractice that surrounds the placing of medicinal products on the market. It is more serious than that because it lies in the conceptual errors made by modern medicine, how it evaluates the drugs that it then forces on doctors, who in turn prescribe them to their patients.

As long as medicine refuses to make the individual sufferer the starting point for their evaluation protocols and continues to dissociate them from the disease and ignore them, there will be dozens more Vioxx's and dozens more Mediator's. What's more, the list gets longer every day: antidepressants (Cymbalta®), vaccines (Cervarix®, Gardasil®), antidiabetics (Galvus®, Janumet®, Lantus®, Onglyza®), antiepileptic (Lyrica®) or antithrombotic medicines (Arixtra®), products for correcting hormonal disorders (Intrinsa®) or to reduce tobacco dependence (Champix®), for skin disorders (Roaccutane®), anti-inflammatory drugs (Arcoxia®), antihemorrhagic drugs (Multaq®), immune-suppressives (Orencia®), anti-osteoporotic medication (Protelos®), for treating dermatitis (Protopic®), and many other products, including anticancer drugs.

All these are under surveillance and some have already been withdrawn from the market.

Integrative medicine offers new perspectives

Faced with the problems that have been brought about by taking a purely analytical approach towards human beings, as part of the process that reinvented the physician as a technician, wouldn't medicine benefit from broadening its outlook and reintegrating the part into the whole? Whether they be cases of acute or chronic illness, an integrative approach always considers the totality of the patient, and places them at the heart of the clinical evaluation, and offers clear and truthful perspectives to everybody involved. The integrative approach that we are proposing gives all due credit to the benefits of the analytical approach where it has been so able at shedding light on the *mechanisms* of disease. Where it falls short is in reaching an understanding of the upstream *agents* and *causes* of disease and the downstream *symptoms* that are peculiar to every individual.

Historically, the comprehensive, multifactorial and integrative approach had always been employed in experimental physiology but this has not been transmitted as one might have expected into clinical medicine, as science was too preoccupied with research into the infinitely small.

This need to synthesize a model that would have as its aim the incorporation of cellular events with all the systems in the entire human being,[20] in other words to develop a truly integrative theory, has parallels with the attempt by physicists to develop a Grand Unified Theory in which the nature of the infinitely small atom is coherent with the infinitely large cosmos, a pursuit that is recognized by everybody as a fruitful challenge.

We trust that it is possible to achieve such a synthesis in our day. Endobiogeny has all the elements of a coherent, detailed and consistent theory that is based entirely on modern scientific data and is capable of responding to this much-needed comprehensive clinical approach.

The advantage of a synthetic approach

Analytical approach to the disease and treatment
Analytical diagnosis ⇒ Disease
⇒ Symptom
Analytical treatment ⇒ Drug dealing with the symptom
In this approach, the individual's terrain has been entirely overlooked

Synthetic approach of the sick, the disease and the treatment
Synthetic diagnosis ⇒ Disease
⇒ Symptom
⇒ Patient
Synthetic treatment ⇒ Integrated treatment of the patients
and their illness
The specificity of the individual's terrain has been comprehensively considered

CHAPTER THREE

A true terrain-based medicine: a new hope for patients

Prevent, treat, cure

What is the terrain?

Let us take the example of three members of the same family who develop hepatitis-A from seafood-poisoning. Why does one get better right away, the second have prolonged jaundice and the third need hospitalization and remains in a critical condition for months?

As another hypothetical example: four women, all faced with the death of a child, will each respond differently to the trauma of this personal tragedy. Why is it that one will fall into a deep depression, the second will immediately stop menstruating, the third will develop breast cancer after a few months, while the last will remain in reasonably good health?

A third example: two men with apparently the same cancer of the prostate are undergoing identical surgical and chemotherapy treatment. Why is one of them totally cured while the other goes on to develop metastases in the bone and dies within 2 years? How can we explain these different outcomes?

The only plausible explanation is given by the condition of their terrain. Medical science defines the terrain as "the set of genetic, physiological, tisssular or humoral factors specific to an individual, which favor the occurrence of a disease or determines its prognosis" (Larousse). This definition of the terrain explains the reason for such different outcomes in the very similar situation that each member of any sample finds themselves.

However important the concept of terrain may be, it remains somewhat vague and is often invoked when one is unable to satisfactorily alter the course of a disease, by blaming it on the terrain rather than admit defeat: "There is nothing to be done; it is your terrain," or when you haven't got a clue: "There is no doubt that it is down to your terrain," rather than to make a well-formulated analysis of a particular physiological state.

The human being cannot be reduced to a simple, unrelated assemblage of functions and organs. It is an autonomous living entity, complete in itself, which reacts and responds continuously as a coherent whole and must constantly adapt to the world. However, as we discussed in a previous chapter, modern medicine has fragmented the body into its multiple components. In neglecting to place each of them in its complex relations with the rest, it has lost the capability of establishing a comprehensive diagnosis of the patient's condition. It is high time that we reclaimed that capability and so have developed a medical approach which *does* take into consideration the relationships unify the local with the global and which allows for a truly integrative and scientific vision of the patient to be established: this is what we mean when we refer to the Endobiogenic approach to the terrain.

The infinite complexity of the human body

Given that our bodies are made up of a myriad number of cells and functions, and tissues and organs, how are they able to operate and cooperate in such a seamless manner that makes our lives what they are? What are the laws that ensure its smooth functioning from the lowest level, the gene, up to the human body as a whole?

Like Russian dolls placed one inside another, each level of the body—from gene to chromosome, from chromosome to nucleus, from nucleus to cell, from cell to organ, from organ to the human body—has its own particular mechanisms, but these are integrated and controlled at a higher level and, in the final analysis by the whole ensemble of the entire organism.

If there is a dysregulation at one level, it is important to identify what it was that generated the dysregulation upstream and understand how it will in turn affect events that are downstream from it. So we should not disassociate the situation at the dysregulated level from all of the other levels nor should we fail to take into account the relationships that connect them, as does the analytical approach of conventional medicine.

For that reason, the careful analysis of each of the mechanisms operating at a given level, in the cell for example, must always be augmented by the study of the mechanisms at work at every other level: the tissue, the organ and the whole body, striving to uncover the relationships that bind them together.

Given the complexity of the human body, we must search for the general physiological rules so that we can understand how a unique functioning individual, who thinks, loves, and stays in balance, can emerge from a system made up of an infinitude of parts. To coin a phrase, how does life live.

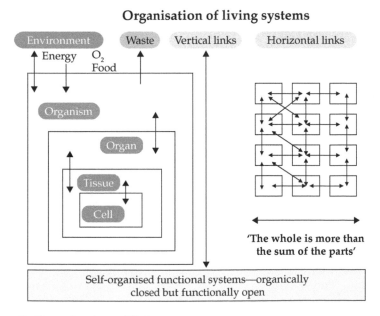

Figure 2: Organization of living systems.

The human body: the whole is more than the sum of its parts

The human body is a complex system made up of parts (organs) that are in turn made up of other parts (tissues). These parts can in turn be broken down into increasingly smaller parts—the cell, with its nucleus which contains the genetic material—each functioning based on very precise laws. From an analytical standpoint, it is convenient, even desirable, to study each part in isolation, to study in detail how each functional unit operates and organizes itself.

But it is a great error to then overlook the relationships that unite each part to the assemblage to which it belongs, and each assemblage to the whole system in which, in turn, it is included. To do so prevents us from arriving at any comprehensive synthesis. By ignoring the local functional relationships within one part, and the functional links that connect it to the larger segment to which it belongs (for example, the gene in relation to the cell, or a cell within an organ and that to the body as a whole) generates the very difficulties that beset modern medicine in its approach to disease. This fragmented approach spawns the profusion of specialties, with an attendant loss of any unifying vision. It leads inevitably to devising treatments that are targeted exclusively on symptoms, and to a management strategy founded on a theory of specific etiology.

The properties of any given system are different and greater to the sum of its functional parts.

What is life?

Life is the succession of an unquantifiable number of physiological phenomena in perpetual movement. Each millisecond, our body destroys millions of cells and rebuilds an equal number of new ones. By these continual processes, the body is thus able to maintain its structure in a functional state, to resist aggressions and any damage so caused, ensuring maintenance and repair at every level of the organism.

For all this to be work smoothly and in harmony, each of the elements that make up who we are must remained in permanent mutual communication. This infinitely complex living system that constitutes our body has to manage and coordinate these relationships, so connecting the cell to the organ, the organ to all the other organs with all the functions that unite them.

Without such coordination, this great symphony of life that allows us to live and carry on living, would be an orchestra without a conductor, as it were, and chaos and disorder would immediately ensue and break down would soon follow. Life cannot be maintained without consistency and purpose ensuring the harmonious operation of cells and organs, so maintaining equilibrium within our bodies.

We need the keys to an understanding of how these relationships bring together all the various elements of the human body so that we can correctly interpret the working of these networks of bodily functions that we can justly call the terrain. There is a directing and coordinating network, and it is the formulation of this system of systems that constitutes the model we propose, which we have named Endobiogeny. These are hypotheses founded entirely on current scientific knowledge. The Endobiogenic approach to the terrain postulates that it is managed by the endocrine system and is based on the recognition of the vital and indispensable role of the hormonal system at all the levels of the human body. Undeniably, this system manages the metabolism, which is nothing less than the permanent and dynamic sequence which commences with catabolism (the breaking down of material), and proceeds to synthesis and reconstruction, which is the anabolic arm. These phenomena are in constant motion, taking place every second throughout our bodies.

It is the only system that penetrates every part of the body, reacting and responding to every type of sensory, metabolic, or physiological demand. Omnipresent and interdependent, connected to all of the other systems, the endocrine system is the only structure that is capable, at least so far as we know from our current knowledge of physiology, to ensure the regulation of life at the level of each element of the human body, and at the same time, to manage itself, which makes it the true manager of the entire living system, the whole of our body.

If the body were a house, its architect would be the endocrine system

The hormonal system begins to operate from the early stages of the development of the embryo, well before the other structures are in place, even before the nervous system develops. This pervasive hormonal coordinator is therefore at work as soon as life begins. It continues to organize itself progressively into a complex system, developing in parallel with the diverse systems and organs as they appear, and which

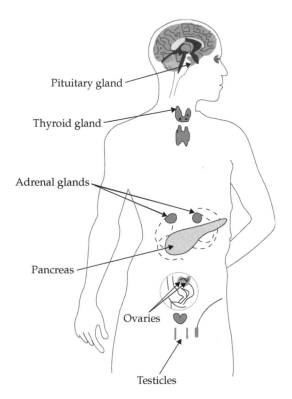

Figure 3: Simplified diagram of the human body.

will eventually constitute the definitive human body of which it will effectively emerge as the sole manager.

This system is very structured and functions according to very precise rules. It is tiered from top to bottom, starting from the hypothalamus to the pituitary gland, from where, by way of the hormones it secretes, the function of the peripheral endocrine glands is controlled. These in their turn secrete other hormones that are distributed throughout by blood and body fluids to their targets, the receptors located on the surface of cells whose operation they will thus control.

Medical physiology has elucidated the effects these hormones have on the cells and organs they reach. They are like messengers carrying information to all levels of the body and so control the entire human body. Although the nucleus of each cell carries all human information within the genome, only certain functions are expressed according to its specialization: a liver cell and a kidney cell play different roles, for example. Each cell must operate in a precise manner and accomplish its

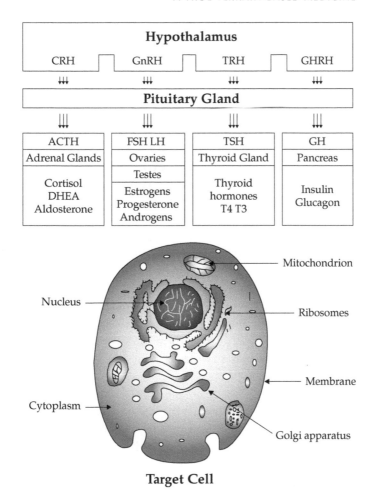

Hypothalamus			
CRH	GnRH	TRH	GHRH
↓↓↓	↓↓↓	↓↓↓	↓↓↓

Pituitary Gland			
↓↓↓	↓↓↓	↓↓↓	↓↓↓
ACTH	FSH LH	TSH	GH
Adrenal Glands	Ovaries	Thyroid Gland	Pancreas
Cortisol DHEA Aldosterone	Testes / Estrogens Progesterone Androgens	Thyroid hormones T4 T3	Insulin Glucagon

Target Cell

Figure 4: The endocrine system.

specific task in a particular order, which usually involves the elaboration of certain proteins.

How does it actually work?

To maintain equilibrium at all levels of the whole system, the hormonal architect must ensure that the entire body functions smoothly and coherently and that all levels from cells to organs operate in harmony with each other and with the whole. In some ways, it acts somewhat like an architect who already knows the plans of our body. It intervenes from moment to moment to maintain connections between different areas of the edifice, to bring material to wherever the need for building arises, to ensure the influx and efflux of provisions, to protect against adverse weather conditions, to repair the house when it is damaged, and to remove waste materials. It plays all the vital roles.

If there is a dearth of material, or there is a hitch in the delivery of material, or if there is some design error, the house will not be functional and, lacking all stability will be rendered uninhabitable. In the same way, the hormonal architect must make all the correct decisions and enact the necessary corrections. As it has to manage a number of specialty trades at the same time, (all the various organs to continue with the construction metaphor), it must make sure that all the tradesmen cooperate and work well together. Otherwise, one or more manufacturing defects will soon put in an appearance and so endanger the whole building.

Let's now use the example of a factory as an analogy of the dynamic way in which the human body functions and the possible reasons for its breakdown. The endocrine system is the factory manager.

The production lines that give rise to the finished product may malfunction from time to time, either gradually or suddenly.

In the case of a gradual malfunction in the production line, the mechanisms may:

- Overreact and hyper-function: giving rise to diseases of excess
  - Immunity dysfunction: Autoimmunity, Allergies
  - Hyper-function of the thyroid gland: Graves' disease
  - Heart: tachycardia

or:

- Slow down and stop: giving rise to diseases of deficiency
  - Diabetes: reduce insulin sensitivity
  - Multiple sclerosis: reduce nerve covering (myelin)

or:

- Gradually grind to a halt: chronic, degenerative disorders
  - Cancers
  - Alzheimer's Dementia
  - Heart disease

The resulting fault may be localized and violently strike a production line element, such as a myocardial infarction in the heart, or a hemorrhagic stroke in the brain. If the manager is able to give the workers the correct orders for immediate repairs, then even a violent crisis may be resolved.

How rapidly the repair will proceed will depend upon the previous state of the factory, whether it was basically in good health. But if the previous state was very poor (unhealthy lifestyle or chronic stress), the repair will take much longer, depending on the number and severity of previous accidents. Sometimes, some production lines are suspended and the management is obliged to implement some maneuver that will bypass the fault and so allow the work of the factory to continue, at a slower pace, if need be.

Likewise, the body may move to exclude an organ that has become harmful to the whole by creating a barrier of fibrous tissue to isolate it from the rest of the body and take it out of the loop, so as to minimize the possible risk for the rest of the body.

For example, in the early stages of infective hepatitis, fibrosis will develop in the liver is an attempt to stop the spread of the virus, but if the fibrosis continues unabated, what was a safeguarding mission could turn against the patient himself. So, this desperate measure, if continued disproportionately, can develop into cirrhosis which, by fighting to preserve life in an effort to protect the liver from death by virus could lead eventually to the death of entire body.

If one of the departments of the factory, which is indispensable to the survival of the whole, becomes suddenly blocked, the whole factory closes down in an instant and will result in the complete standstill, which is death. This is why an apparently healthy person can die within minutes of a sudden obstruction in a coronary artery causing a massive myocardial infarction.

In a car assembly plant, there is a plan for the organization of the production lines to ensure that the work is carried out in a consistent and rigorous manner: one step after another, in the correct sequence. If any step is omitted, the car produced will be abnormal. The same is true for the human body.

The succession of sequences that ensures the demolition and reconstruction of cells, allowing life to be maintained and renewed, is very precise ordered. If this order is not respected, all sorts of problems will arise. It is this order and these rules that were brought to light by Endobiogeny, and which we will now go on to explain further.

*The key to understanding the hormonal sequences
governing our body*

Although modern medical physiology demonstrates a profound understanding of the effects of hormones on the organs and tissues of the
body, and those functions in which they are instrumental, it has yet to
propose a coherent and integrated system to elucidate the commands
and sequences by which the endocrine system operates.

The Endobiogenic system puts forward a unique integrative view of
the functioning of the human body and shows how the connections are
made at all levels of its structures and functions. It was conceived by
Dr. Christian Duraffourd, with whom I worked for over 35 years, and
this book the first to explain its workings for the general reader.

This new approach builds on knowledge derived from the analytical
sciences, but integrates it into an inclusive and dynamic view of the
individual. The malfunction of one part can only be interpreted in the
context of the harmonized operation of the whole, and must always
be analyzed in relation to the whole body.

We have already made the case for life to be considered as a permanent
progression of an alternating series of destruction and reconstruction.
The understanding of the order in which these sequences are carried
out is crucial, because it allows one to see why and how the disruptions
of the normal operation of the endocrine system can contribute to an
explanation of all disease processes in the new light of these integrated
and comprehensive mechanisms.

The logic of these sequences is inferred from the operation of the four
endocrine axes. Medical science teaches us that there are four major
endocrine axes according to which we can classify each hormone based
on its origin and its mode of action. Let us now define the hormones
based on these axes and see how these axes work, how each of them
is connected with each of the others, and into what sequence they are
set in motion. We should bear in mind that these axes are sending
instructions to every cell in the body; the way that these the orders are
sent and received will has influence their mode of operation.

The **corticotropic axis** is activated first. It has a catabolic function,
which means that overall it breaks down and releases material. It secretes
cortisol from the outer layer of the gland and releases adrenaline from
the inner part. These two make energy immediately available in the
form of glucose, so that the body can cope with the whatever challenges
it faces.

After this first, very rapid catabolic stage in which material is released and made available as energy, the metabolic process is completed by the mobilization of the axis which delivers proteins; these have already been built: they were manufactured by the anabolic processes located in the **gonadotropic axis**.

If this second axis is to respond to the call from the first and proceed with all its activities, it will require more sustained energy. This is provided by the **thyrotropic axis**, which is catabolic and will obtain this additional energy from the breakdown of lipids and particularly from cholesterol.

Finally, the reconstruction axis is set in motion. This will ensure that all the elements that were previously broken down are now reconstructed and put in place. This anabolic role is performed by the **somatotropic axis** by the hormone insulin, and insulin-like growth factors. This fourth axis completes and closes the cycle.

Whenever a person faces any type of aggression or challenge, whether it be physical, mental, social or emotional, the energetic material of his or her body must be mobilized. We have an alert or vigilance system to

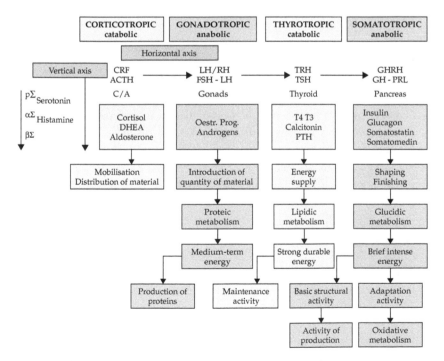

Figure 5: The four endocrine axes and their functional purpose.

recognize if such an attack is imminent: it is one of the many functions of the *autonomic nervous system*. It is the first to react and immediately triggers the cascade of hormonal reactions that permits us to respond to the aggression.

To do this, the patient needs immediate energy, which requires the setting in motion of the system that mobilizes material to be made available to the body (see the diagram above).

The reality is very complex because the sequence of reactions carried out in the body involves concomitant vertical, horizontal, and diagonal cycles, involving hormonal carriers, buffer systems and receptors located on the surface of each cell.

The precise knowledge of these mechanisms is important for the doctor who wants to delve deeper into this overarching approach to the dynamic functioning of the human body.[1]

The succession of the four endocrine–metabolic pathways is conducted in the following order:

– catabolism (breaking down, corticotropic axis)
– anabolism (construction, gonadotropic axis)
– catabolism (breaking down, thyrotropic axis)
– anabolism (reconstruction, somatotropic axis)

This very rapid succession of sequences (each millisecond, millions of cells die and an equal number of cells are born) takes place continuously within the human body to provide unbroken maintenance and repair of its structure and its ability to respond to aggression and challenges. This constitutes the very nature of adaptation.

If the steps in this succession are reversed or altered in any way, or if one of them is too intense, or on the contrary, is deficient, or if a step is skipped, the effects at the level of the cell will be immediate. The consequences will be felt sooner or later by the body, depending upon the quality and nature of the imbalance, its intensity, or how prolonged, or poorly adapted.

The fundamental causes of diseases are to be found in the malfunction of the hormonal system. However, in general, modern medicine takes the view that all disease suddenly appears as if by magic, without any preexisting reality. At no time does it consider the various mechanisms leading to this "big bang." It takes a "freeze frame" view of life while, of course, life is an endless reel of film in continuous movement, and the path that any disease follows is necessarily the logical result of the previous events on the strip of film.

With the "big bang," when disease bursts onto the scene, it signifies the existence of a previous, hidden imbalance, a consequence of dysfunctions lurking in the depths of the body, symptom free for some period of time. This hidden period allows the peril to gather its harmful and destructive power: a virus, an excess or shortage of an enzyme, a faulty gene, an unhealthy lifestyle, a change of season, an emotional shock, all *"the heartache and the thousand natural shocks that flesh is heir to"* to quote Shakespeare's Hamlet.

The modern medical approach identifies the body's response to this aggression, whatsoever it might be, as the sole cause of the disease but the response is in fact fundamentally dependent on the state of the terrain of the person who experiences the aggression.

The biology of functions: a tool that reveals the hidden imbalances in the body

Based on simple straightforward principles

Doctors routinely take blood from their patients either just as a general check-up or to investigate whether the symptoms presented might presage the arrival of some new disorder. The test results are interpreted as normal if they fall within a defined range or, conversely, lie above or below that range. For example, to exclude or to verify a diagnosis of diabetes, the patient's blood is checked for its glucose levels along with a corroborating test performed on the red cells (called a hemoglobin A1c). If these are both elevated the diagnosis of diabetes is confirmed, and the doctor will then prescribe medication to reduce blood glucose levels. Another reason for taking blood is to monitor the progression in a disease where the diagnosis has already been established, for example inflammatory markers or liver enzymes need to be monitored in many conditions, including liver disease. This is the modern approach of biology: it establishes a direct link between the levels measured in the blood, identifies the disease, and establishes the treatment of choice.

The Biology of Functions is somewhat different. The taking of a blood sample for the Biology of Functions is identical to any clinical setting, but the interpretation of the results seeks a deeper understanding than is provided by the conventional analysis of blood test results.

It is a question of extracting more information from the results that are reported to the doctor by the laboratory. The main idea is based on a principle that is actually quite straightforward: *that which is found within the circulating blood is nothing more than the consequence of what the organism was manufacturing.*

Let us take red blood cells and white blood cells as an example. It is entirely a routine matter to count the number of red cells and white cells in the patient's blood and is perfectly straightforward. But instead of limiting the analysis to only these levels, as is the conventional medical practice, the Biology of Functions looks to evaluate those elements that contributed to the production of red and white blood cells.

Physiology, which is an essential science in a doctor's training, teaches us that these cells are manufactured in specialized tissue within the bone marrow, under the predominant action of androgens (male hormones) for red blood cells and estrogens (female hormones) for the white blood cells. It follows from this that we can take the number of red cells and white cells in the circulating blood of a patient to tell us what kind of effect his or her androgens and estrogens are having on the tissues of the body in question. By doing this, we are looking upstream of the circulating blood. In other words, the hormones are upstream. The tissue—the bone marrow in this example—is midstream. The quantified output of red and white cells by the marrow is downstream. Thus, we have a causal chain of events in the flow of life: cause (hormone), action (blood cell production in the marrow), effect (change in the number of red and white blood cells).

After understanding this, we can go further. By establishing a relationship between the number of red cells and the number of white cells present in the blood, we get a simple index that we have named the "Genital ratio." It allows the doctor to assess the *relative* activity of his or her male hormones at tissue level compared with the female hormones, according to the following formula: red blood cells divided by white blood cells, and the relationship between the androgen activity and estrogen activity. The higher this index, the stronger is the tissue-level effects of androgens compared with that of estrogens (cf. tables in Chapter 5). The lower this index, the stronger is the tissue-level effects of estrogens compared with that of androgens.

Let us now move on to the next stage which examines the different *types* of white blood cell. The full blood count (FBC) of a patient includes what is known as a differential white cell count (WBC) and platelet count. White blood cells are not all the same: they constitute a family of five different types of selves. They were named by their ability to take up different stains and forms part of the history of microscopy. Let's start with one of the five types which go by the name of eosinophils. Eosinophils play a crucial role in symptoms of allergy. The higher the number of eosinophils, the more severe allergic symptoms tend to be. Moving on to another white cell type: the monocytes. They are important immune agents in the protection of the human body from infection. The higher the number of monocytes found in the full blood count, the more severe inflammatory phenomena tend to be.

Decades of scientific research in physiology have demonstrated that the number of eosinophils in the blood increases when the hormone ACTH (the hormonal response to aggression) is secreted. When it comes to monocytes, research has shown a correlation between their numbers and the anabolic hormone from the gonadic axis called follicle stimulating hormone, or FSH. By calculating the ratio between the number of eosinophils and monocytes in the circulating blood, we obtain a new index, called the "Adaptation index." The ratio eosinophils/monocytes allows the doctor to evaluate the *relative* activity of ACTH compared with that of the hormone FSH at the tissue level.

The higher the index, the greater the ACTH activity compared with that of FSH; the lower the index, the higher the FSH activity compared with that of ACTH. This can provide useful guidance on how the patient's body manages its response to stress.

I have often seen patients who have a very high level of ACTH activity, which demonstrates the degree to which they secrete this hormone in response to the challenges they face. It also gives you some idea of the degree of alertness and the requisite mobilization of energy made always available to their bodies: these patients are in a state equivalent to that resulting from going quietly about their daily business when suddenly faced by a tiger on the corner of the street.

The biology of functions: mapping the terrain

Thus, starting from a simple blood test comprising a dozen or so standard biomarkers, such as full blood count with platelets, the proportion of certain enzymes, and other specified items, we can elaborate a system of interconnected algorithms, all according to recognized physiological data. This system generates many more indexes than those already mentioned. This considerable amount of data provides a broader understanding of the biological phenomena at work within the body than the purely analytical approach currently in use. We have named this system the Biology of Functions.[2]

This complex system was conceived by Dr. Christian Duraffourd when working as Research Associate at the General Surgery and Oncology Clinic of Boucicaut Hospital, from 1989 to 1996 in the Department led by Professor Jacques Reynier. This groundbreaking work led us establish some 172 indexes, each one related to an endocrine or metabolic activity, or a tissue state or a degree of responsiveness. Examples include cell necrosis, insulin resistance, bone remodeling, immunity, oxidative stress, the potential for the development of abnormal cells. These indexes allow us to capture the state of the individual's structure and the way in which he or she reacts to stressors and so represents the status of his or her terrain.

This integrative approach to physiology and biology, which is inexpensive compared to tissue biopsies, ultrasounds and MRI scans, provides use with a significant amount of new information. It allows the clinician to evaluate the state of the patient's terrain with specific numerical values and follows these values over time to objectively evaluate the capabilities of their body. We have seen that the endocrine system is the architect in charge of the human body's function.

It is important to understand that by superimposing these indexes on the diagram of axes above (Figure 4: The endocrine axes), we can create a map that precisely quantifies hormonal activity, and so gives us a much more complete overview of the way in which the patient's body works, from the cellular and tissular level, via the vital organs, right up to a global view of the whole organism.

This map gives us a detailed snapshot of the current state of a patient's structure, rather like a physiological identity card from which you can read the basic resting state, but also the functional capacity to respond to self-generated stress and to deal with and adapt to the outside world.

The mapping starts with the first consultation, and provides real benefits for patient and doctor alike, because it gives them both objective, quantified data on the state of the terrain.

Following the evolution of a patient's indexes over the course of treatment is one of its most useful features. It affords the clinician an insight into the inbuilt tendencies of an individual's terrain, and so guides the therapeutic choices in an accurate manner which will be modified according to the developments in the terrain. It also allows the impact of any type of treatment to be measured. Whether treatment is by synthetic molecules or by medicinal plants or other natural products, its effectiveness can be judged objectively.

Over the course of 20 years, more than 30,000 Biology of Functions have been performed for patients of all ages with all types of diseases and in all manner of states of health. Around the world, first in France, and then across Europe, the Americas and North Africa, general practitioners and specialists have used this marvelous tool to support their patients (see Chapter 7 "The Growing International Influence of Clinical Phytotherapy" and Chapter 9 "Carol's Case: Metastatic Breast Cancer").

We believe that this innovative resource should be made available to all patients and not just to the few. Further, we are convinced that it will open new perspectives onto our understanding of the mechanisms involved in the genesis of degenerative and cardiovascular disease, as well as metabolic and immune disorders. We published the results of our research several years ago and we asked the French scientific authorities if they would authorize the use of this system in our hospitals. We are still waiting for their response.

Fortunately, this work is carried on elsewhere and an international network is being created of practitioners and researchers who are aware that taking the terrain into account will help them take better care of their patients' health.

Things we can learn from an index

The following example shows the wealth of information provided by the simple examination of one of the indexes of the Biology of Functions. (Paper presented by Dr. Lapraz at a World Health Organization symposium on medicinal plants, on October 17, 2003 in Tunis.)

The histamine index, obtained from a blood count, allows one to evaluate, thanks to certain algorithms, the activity of the histamine at tissue level, without a direct count of histamine in the serum.

After a chemotherapy infusion, patients may present with significant allergic-type reactions in the digestive tract, or the skin, or elsewhere. The chemical mediator responsible for these types of reactions is histamine.

Mrs. Annie C., born on December 4, 1954, underwent cancer surgery on June 19, 2002 for an adenocarcinoma of her right breast at the Georges Pompidou European Hospital of the Paris Public Hospital System.

Postoperatively, she was administered six cycles of chemotherapy with Adriamycin (86.5 mg), Ifosfamide (1,165 mg) and Taxotere

(130 mg), within BCIRG-005 Protocol (Dates: August 8, 2002; August 29, 2002; September 19, 2002; October 10, 2002; October 31, 2002; November 21, 2002). She received no other treatment; in particular, neither cortisone nor bone marrow stimulating agents were administered.

Let us look at the evolution of the index of histamine during the treatment.

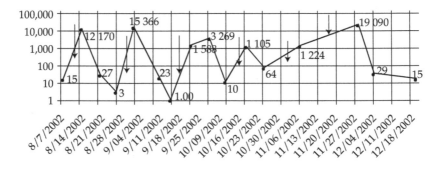

The arrows indicate the time when the chemotherapy was administered. On the diagram showing the evolution of the histamine index, we see a surge of histamine activity in the days following the treatment, which appears to drop in eight to ten days and return to the baseline state. Thus, the index which, before the first chemotherapy on August 7, 2002 was 15, surges to 12,170, seven days after the chemotherapy infusion, and goes down to 3 on August 28.

Her body's response curve after each infusion is the same: a significant rise in the histamine response after the infusion, then a gradual drop and return to the baseline state. At the last infusion, the histamine surge is even stronger reflecting the fact that over time, the allergic response to the injected chemotherapy has become increasingly severe. This shows that her tolerance of the treatment is progressively decreasing, which may, therefore, compromise its continuation.

Based on the intensity and the rapidity of onset of the histamine peak and its decline, it is easier to predict the likelihood of the patient presenting with strong histamine-related reactions such as nausea, vomiting, headache, or other allergies. With the insight gained from the index, the appropriate complementary therapy can be chosen to allow the patient to tolerate the chemotherapy better, and thus help her continue with it.

This monitoring of one simple index shows that it is possible to introduce new perspectives into medical practice for the follow-up of the patients, regardless of the type of disease they suffer from.

The Biology of Functions currently includes 172 indexes, each providing essential information. The interrelated indexes provide a panoramic view of the structural and functional condition of the patient and his or her potential risk of developing a disease. It allows the development of his or her terrain to be monitored, differentiating intrinsic fluctuations from a reaction to a treatment.

A new perspective on medicine that makes prevention possible

If we accept that a healthy state consists of finding the best possible point of balance for any individual, it is a good starting point for understanding how disease may come about.

Faced with difficulties and challenges or shocks, whether external, for example: facing sudden cold or the shock of sudden loss, eating tainted food, taking a poorly tolerated medicine, facing stress at work; or stress coming from within, which might include a genetic disorder, an enzymatic abnormality, or hyperactivity of a hormone triggering an autoimmune disease, the body will necessarily have to react. It will have to face the aggression and somehow "digest" it.

The body will have to prepare a physiological response to confront the aggressor, depending upon its nature and its pathogenicity.[3] In other words, it will have to mobilize the appropriate physiological mechanisms and elements and transport them to where the aggression is located, thereby enabling the body to fight it off. These mechanisms include local congestion, inflammation and the delivery of immune factors. If the body is strong enough and well prepared, it will defeat and eliminate the aggressor. The reaction that the body has mounted to the aggression, having no reason to persist, will come to a halt and so the body will return to its previous state and will be healed.

On the other hand, if for one reason or another, allied to the basic state of the individual person, the body's response is disproportionate to the aggression, or it falters before completion, or it is poorly adapted, it will no longer be able to mount a correct or adequate defense against the aggressor. A pathological imbalance will have been set up, and this may well evolve into a permanent state of imbalance, and that is when disease is likely to take hold. The crucial point is therefore the ability of the body, or its incapacity, to return to its basal physiological state that existed before the aggression.

The medicine of today concerns itself only with disease, but the manifestation of disease is but the tip of the iceberg. It fails to accord due significance to those hidden depths in the ocean of physiology: the terrain. Medical science has developed an immense body of knowledge about the pathophysiology of disease but, by restricting itself to the abnormal mechanisms of established disease, it ignores the study of the physiological state that preceded in disease. From our perspective as Endobiogenists, it is precisely the state of the terrain prior to the onset of the imbalance, unique to each person that allows us to understand the characteristics of the disease in each person. This can help us understand why, in any particular case, a disease can be moderate or severe, isolated or diffuse, acute or chronic, more or less responsive to treatment in one patient versus another. Hence, we return to our observation that we must always contextualize the disease to the state of the whole person.

The integrative approach in medicine

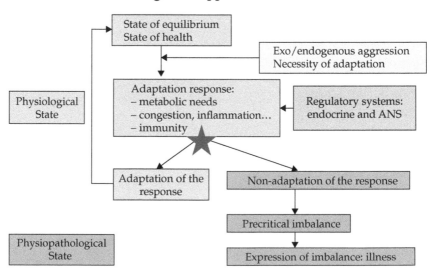

Figure 6: Integrative vision in medical practice.

In its approach to the disease, conventional medicine positions itself just after this breaking point (the star on the diagram) where the individual is no longer in a normal physiological state; he or she falls ill, and the disease establishes its own pathological mechanisms of development and evolution.

This explains why two brothers living in the same house and infected by the same streptococcus bacterium will present with illnesses that progress in two very different ways. One will develop catarrhal tonsillitis that will be responsive to treatment, and the other will suffer several relapses and will go on to develop acute rheumatic fever. Just as in a pine forest with dry undergrowth and trees with inflammable oils, fire spreads much faster than in woodland composed of mature trees where the deep shade limits regeneration of the undergrowth.[4] Likewise, someone with a terrain akin flammable undergrowth, will be at greater risk of developing a progressive disease compared with someone who does not have such a terrain. Considering the basic physiological state of the individual is therefore essential. It gives us the means to offer a better treatment for the illness while at the same time to support the ill person by correcting the underlying state of the terrain. But more than this, it enables us to practice truly preventative medicine by identifying the hidden imbalances that preceded the onset of the disease.

The endobiogenic timeline

It is of the greatest importance for a doctor to spend time with a patient so as to collect the maximum information on the medical history. It is an essential first step in the doctor-patient relationship.

Time to listen

The doctor task on taking on a new patient is to listen and record relevant information for the follow-up. As current medical practice accords so little time for a consultation, generally, the doctor writes a brief history of the major events in the patient's medical life, past diseases and any surgical interventions, and assesses the family history for potential risks for any particular disease. This data is very important, of course, but terrain-based medicine requires collection and recording of much more detailed information.

It is not enough just to note the name of the disease and its particular form, with viral hepatitis, for instance, whether A, B or C. We need to record accurately the chronology events and relate them to other conditions or symptoms, make a detailed description of its progression as well as the associated signs, clarify its relation with the subject's environment and lifestyle (diet, socio-professional, emotional life, etc.) and note in particular the response to any treatment, because each sign, as innocuous as it may seem, will help us identify the physiological connections underlying the disease.

All this detailed information recorded on a timeline from birth up to the date of the first consultation allows us to create a physiological profile from the "patient's story" and to begin to understand the condition of his or her terrain from an early stage.

For example, a case of simple non-purulent acne in a 9-year-old girl does not arise from the same physiological abnormalities as the sudden appearance of purulent acne in on the face and upper back of a 15-year-old boy. The difference between the physiological anomalies in these two cases points to the particular state of each individual terrain. If they are followed-up later in life similar, the same kind of analysis will give the doctor a better understanding of how their endocrine system works and, rather like a detective, will begin to make connections that will help the person recognize their signs come to a better understanding of the manner in which their terrain works.

Conducting the clinical examination

This examination will be based on the same principles: not missing anything, examining everything, taking everything into account and relating signs one to another to better understand what their true significance is. We will illustrate in the next chapter how important it is to devote time to the patient during every consultation, even if the doctor has known the patient for years.

Writing the prescription

This is approached in the same way. We establish a plan of action that considers the disease and the patient *as a complete ensemble*.

The endobiogenic approach contrasted with conventional medicine: two ways of providing care

We will now present three cases to illustrate the differences between Endobiogeny and the conventional approach towards the disease and the care of the sick.

1: A child with recurrent ear infections

The mother of this 5-years-old boy brought in to see me in 1997 gave me a copy of her child's medical records so that I could appreciate how complex his case had become. The records had been scrupulously filled out by successive general practitioners and specialists who conscientiously recorded their diagnosis and the treatment prescribed after each consultation. They made quite surprising reading.

We start with his first ear infection (Otitis media) in November, 1992, when he was aged seven months. Since that time, he had been taken for examination on no fewer than 42 occasions for the very same reason: recurrent ear infections! Over the 4 years that preceded our meeting, a variety of problems had afflicted this child's ears, ranging from pain to acute otitis media. A range of conditions were confirmed by otoscope examination and a litany of terms was duly recorded: scarring, congestion, inflammation, perforated drums, serous or serous-bullous or serous-congestive otitis media, with or without effusion, unilateral or bilateral. All faithfully reported.

All treatments were also carefully documented: ten types of antibiotics had been prescribed 38 times. Over 4 years he had received a total of ten months of daily antibiotics, administered morning and evening! In addition to this, he was prescribed corticosteroids eight times for three consecutive months, plus 37 prescriptions for antitussives and a number of anti-inflammatories prescribed over the long-term. All of these treatments were completely in accord with the standards of care established by the relevant medical authorities.

What should we make of this kind of situation?

This example, extreme as it is, is by no means exceptional. The use of very powerful medicinal products for trivial complaints has become so commonplace that the doctors have lost sight of the risks to their patients. This culture of trivialization is entrenched and institutionalized by public agencies that demand mothers to have their children "correctly" treated, "or to keep them home because their runny nose will spread germs to the other children in nursery school." It has become normal to have infants on "prophylactic" antibiotics for two or three months, to avoid infections over the winter. But what will be the consequences of this excessive use?

How can we not question the costs incurred by children in the long run when they are subjected to such potent and extensive chemical aggression? How can the development of these little ones not be affected as they grow up, by having their organism unduly and repetitively tampered with? Should we not be troubled at seeing an increasing number of children with debilitating conditions and that these can sometimes trigger diseases that are far from being trivial?

Should we not protect our children from this chemical pollution to which they are subjected by the repeated administration of powerful treatments for conditions that do not require such interventions, and which can be treated by other means?

What is the solution?

Before discussing the case of this child, we might clarify the nature of his condition. Otitis media is an organ disease affecting the ear, or to be more precise, the eardrum. It is a chronic inflammatory condition. In most cases, this inflammation is an exaggerated response that sensitizes the immune cells in the region of the ear. The doctors who treated this little boy perfectly examined the affected organ that gave rise to the symptoms, but they didn't go any further than this observation.

Now, the normal physiological functioning of the ear requires the autonomic nervous system to ensure the smooth movements of the Eustachian tube, which allows the ear to communicate with the nose and throat. It also relies on the hormonal system to supervise the state of the immune system.

His autonomic nervous system is first in line to mount a robust defense against an aggressor, in this case a microbe close to the eardrum. By blocking the internal orifice of the Eustachian tube, the sympathetic branch of the autonomic system will initiate and maintain local congestion, which will in turn create favorable conditions for the germ to be nourished, and so multiply.

We should then consider the role of the endocrine system that is engaged in combat with the inflammation and in maintaining a good state of local immunity. And so, the doctor will move from investigating the ear drum towards the other organs involved in managing the immune response, such as the thymus, spleen and liver, which are part of the more general defense system.

A full clinical examination of the child revealed that these various systems were out of balance, as was his thyroid. It is known to play a key role in the formation of the tonsils and other local lymph nodes. In the case of this boy, his thyroid played a significant role in the chronicity of his infected ear. Also, his pancreas, overly stressed by an excessive consumption of sweets, may have predisposed him to repeated infections.

Accordingly, any treatment must take into consideration this child's entire body, not just the state of his ear. A whole-body treatment requires a multi-pronged approach, mainly using whole-plant extracts with well-known properties and adapted to the purpose sought[5]:

- sugar-free, dairy free diet, with no snacking between meals to avoid surges of insulin
- pancreatic support with walnut and blackberry
- liver support by drainage, using sapwood of linden and chicory to relieve his overburdened liver from the burden of strong pharmaceutical products
- regulation of the excessive activity of his autonomic system using lavender and thyme
- regulation of his thyroid axis and adrenal gland with extract of oat, pichi, and blackcurrant
- inhalation of essential oils such as pine, eucalyptus, lavender for their antiseptic action

Very soon after these measures and treatments were initiated, the persistent ear infections ceased.

Thus, in the case of otitis, and especially when recurrent, we should not look solely at the eardrum; we must broaden the understanding of the disease and establish the links between the ear and the physiological mechanisms that ensure its regulation, and take measures accordingly.

2: The treatment of a patient with eczema

In this case, we will follow the same approach as for the otitis media. Eczema is considered a lesion exclusive to the skin. However, we know that the microcirculation of blood exercises a significant impact on the skin and that this is under the regulation of the sympathetic branch of the autonomic nervous system. We also know that the fat metabolism plays a large part in this disease and so cannot be disassociated from the state of the liver. Furthermore, it has been demonstrated that emotional stress influences the state of the skin by way of hormonal effects in conjunction with the organs responsible for the assimilation of nutrients. As this is not intended to be a medical treatise, I will not go into further detail. Suffice to say that, based on these simple considerations, it will not be enough for the physician just to prescribe the application of an ointment. On the contrary, clarifying the connections between the liver and the skin together with the emotional state constitute a clinical imperative in every case of eczema.

This research is essential and can only be achieved by a detailed analysis of the patient: it means searching for signs, past and present, to investigate the state of the liver and the nervous system. There are many different reasons for developing eczema, complicated by hormonal or liver problems or emotional stress, so no two treatments will be the same.

This holistic approach explains the often spectacular results that can be obtained by using a medicinal plant to improve the state of a patient's liver. But of course, medical intervention should not be confined to a purely symptomatic level, but should try to identify the real physiological reasons behind this eczema. If we truly want to place Endobiogeny in the service of the patient and if our goal is long-term healing, we should go beyond addressing the symptoms. We must position the patients' liver and mind in the context of their entire life, their lifestyle, their emotional life, and their relationship with others.

Such an approach leads to accountability and the involvement of patients in their own care, and provides them with a clear outlook on their problem. This awareness can only lead to a change in their relationship with the world and with themselves.

Thus, starting with a physical ailment—whatever and wherever it may be—we need in the end to look at its relationship with other organs and the totality of functions, to arrive at an overall, so-called "integrative" medical strategy. This assists the doctor to prioritize the clinical approach beginning with listening and communicating with the patient, then proceeding to a detailed and comprehensive clinical examination, followed by an analysis of data provided by the blood test supplemented by the Biology of Functions indexes, allowing the patient enough time to express conflicts and emotional difficulties. All this will be needed so that a personalized therapeutic strategy, one that is coherent and reliable, to be implemented.

This comprehensive approach towards the terrain opens new pathways for doctors and helps them solve the chronic problems that many patients endure for a long time: chronic colds, migraines, recurrent urinary infections and many other complaints they cannot shake off. The kinds of ailment for which modern medicine has very little to offer.

3: Bronchiolitis in infants and young children

This case will show how seasonal changes can have a significant influence on the outbreak of diseases by modifying the child's metabolism. In its edition of November 3, 2011, the French medical daily newspaper *Le Quotidien du Medecin* highlighted a report issued by the *Institut de veille sanitaire* (Health Watch), that warned of the rapid spread of bronchiolitis among infants in France. This acute inflammation of the bronchioles[6] is a matter of grave public health concern since it affects 460,000 infants per year. The principal culprit for causing this disease has been identified as RSV, which stands of the respiratory syncytial virus.

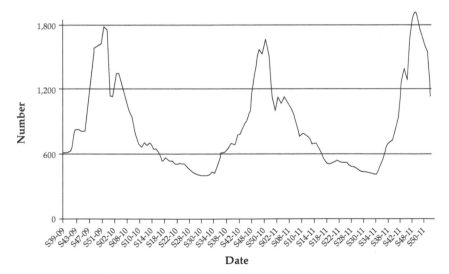

Figure 7: Bronchiolitis.
Number of children under 2 years of age with bronchiolitis seen weekly in the emergency departments of the 170 hospitals participating in the survey since 2009.
Source: September 29, 2011, Institut de Veille Sanitaire.

The conventional conception of this illness is that it is simply the result of the action of a virus attacking the mucous membranes in a child who has somehow picked it up from the environment. Several factors influence the risk of infection, such as being in the care of local authorities, poor quality urban housing, low socio-economic status, passive smoking and many siblings. Preexisting respiratory abnormalities (such as a narrowing of lower airways) and a parental history of asthma as well as prematurity at birth are also contributory factors.

These elements undeniably play a contributory role, but do these factors provide an adequate explanation for this rapid expansion of bronchiolitis, and for its severity in a certain group of children? This question could validly be asked of any infectious disease.

A possible interpretation of seasonal patterns of bronchiolitis

If we examine the number of new cases of bronchiolitis, it is striking that they do not appear, or only very rarely, in the months of April and May and they reach their lowest level at the end of August. From the middle of October, the number of cases we see starts to rise gradually then very rapidly in November, reaching a maximum in December. This explosion of cases in winter shows an increase by a factor of about 1,000. From late January we see a rapid fall in the numbers and then they fall away until, by the end of May there are only a few isolated cases.

How are we to make of this pattern? What are the factors could explain how the immune system of hundreds of thousands of infants has been compromised to such a degree and all at the same time, to the extent that many of them have to be taken hospital, while they were all in apparently good health a month previously? What is going on in the bodies of these children?

The explanation provided by endobiogeny: adaptation to the seasonal changes

We learn from biology that every organism needs to put its mechanisms of adaptation in motion each time it has to cope with change. In August, when summer comes to an end in the Northern hemisphere, the level of our metabolism will no longer be sufficient to negotiate the coming cold season. Migratory birds are equipped with very fine electromagnetic sensors and so can pick up these environmental cues that warn them of the climatic change waiting in the wings. The shortening of the days and changes in the quality of light tells them that it is time for them to leave for warmer climes.

Likewise, we have internal clocks bequeathed to our genes by evolution, which can detect subtle differences in our environment, even if we are not conscious of them. These lead to changes in our bodies that help us adapt to the forthcoming climatic changes and have been validated by large-scale experimental studies. These adaptive changes to the cold of the winter will be translated in our bodies by the resetting of relationships between different parts of our hormonal system. This re programming matches changes in our bodies with changes in the season, a relic of our evolutionary past.

How does the body adapt to seasonal change?

To respond to this need to adapt to fixed and inevitable change, a succession of increased hormonal secretions will gradually take place, according to a very precise sequence. At the end of August, the significant boost in the secretion of cortisol, provider of energy and regulator of the major functions of the body, ensures a progressively increasing level of activity of the thyroid gland, responsible for energy metabolism, and production of body heat. This rise will reach a peak in mid-December and then plateau until the end of January. This phenomenon is genetically programmed and not a matter of personal choice.

Then, towards the end of winter, this increase in thyroid activity will no longer be necessary, and so will gradually decrease to reach its lowest level in the spring, when the adaptation to the cold is no longer required.[7]

What happens when this mechanism seizes up and we get the flu?

The thyroid and the adrenal glands are usually the principle suspects!

In fact, cortisol and the thyroid hormones play an important role in the immune defense of the body in its fight against germs and viruses. Their effectiveness is directly related to the ability of these glands to produce them. Thus, a delayed or blunted hormonal response will result in a weakening of the local defense mechanisms against the bronchiolitis virus. It is this combination of hormones and local immunity that will render a child vulnerable to this external threat.

Why does this disease affect the bronchial tubes
and small airways?

To adapt to seasonal changes, the thyroid needs to be activated for the oxidation of glucose. Oxidation is the burning of sugar within cells to make the energy they need. The currency of this cellular energy is stored in a compound called adenosine triphosphate, or ATP. This oxidation process, like all burning, creates heat, which helps us deal with the cold of winter. Oxidation during the change in the seasons increases the need for oxygen, the second ingredient for releasing energy after glucose. The respiratory system delivers the oxygen needed by the body. Thus, the small bronchial tubes are called upon more in the winter to help bring oxygen into the body. In poorly adapting patients—with an imbalance in adrenal or thyroid function, the bronchioles are over-solicited to compensate for these hormonal shortcomings. From here on in, other changes occur to the point where the small airways become damaged, which makes it easier for the virus to gain a foothold and start an infection.

The contribution that seasonal adaptation makes to the occurrence of peaks in bronchiolitis can be explained by these mechanisms. But the increase in the frequency of this disease in the last few years raises other questions. What is the role of the repeated exposure of children from birth or even in the womb to pharmaceutical agents that alter their immune capabilities? The more antibiotics and steroids given, the *weaker* the immune system becomes and the greater the frequency of infections.

Medical science should therefore give priority to preventative measures for these very young children. This will entail gaining a more precise understanding of the condition of each individual, and then administering treatments that will support rather than be aggressive to their organism. This can be achieved by using whole-plant extracts such as black current buds, for example, as they have outstanding anti-inflammatory properties. The use of steroids should be restricted to absolute emergencies.

In addition, the therapy adopted should offer support to the organs and functions involved in the management of immunity, notably the liver, pancreas, and spleen. It should also strengthen the adaptive capability of their adrenal and thyroid glands, as well as help the autonomic nervous system perform as effectively as possible. Micronutrients with anti-infective activity such as copper, gold and silver should be included in the treatment plan.

It can also be very helpful to reduce the spread of the viruses involved in these infections by the diffusion of solutions of volatile oils both in the home and other places where these infants congregate. Good examples of antiviral essential oils include eucalyptus, lavender, cinnamon, and niaouli. Thousands of scientific works have been conducted around the world, in laboratory and in clinical trials that support this recommendation (for more information, please consult the Bibliography at the end of this book). There are older scientific studies[8] as well that have provided clear clinical evidence.

Preventative treatment options

Bronchiolitis reflects a temporary glitch in the body's struggle to adapt to a challenge. The doctor's primary goal should be to offer preventative measures to ensure that the body is prepared to face the winter months. The last two weeks of August, before the body starts to implement its response to the seasonal changes, is the best time to implement this. The purpose of the Endobiogenic treatment will be to provide the elements that will allow the child's body to respond proportionately to preparation for the shorter and colder months ahead. A careful clinical examination will be needed to identify the vulnerable points, and is a mandatory step before trying to correct them.

The opportunities that medicinal plants can offer are numerous and varied. They are up to the task of meeting the various requirements for preventing this type of disease, and depend upon the needs of each individual case, and are likely to include some or all the following actions:

– **anti-inflammatories** that decrease the intensity of local sensitivity to aggressors: plantain, mallow, great mullein
– **expectorants**, which facilitate the expulsion of bronchial secretions: elecampane, nasturtium, sundew, or sweet violet
– **antispasmodics** that relax the tone in bronchial smooth muscle, making them less likely to collapse: sweet woodruff, field poppy
– **anti-infective agents**, fighting against the frequent risk of superinfections: essential oils of lavender, eucalyptus, Ceylon cinnamon, or myrtle

- **regulators** of the autonomic nervous system, reducing excessive activity of the parasympathetic system and supporting adrenaline in the beta-sympathetic system thereby reducing the need for bronchodilators frequency of administration of salbutamol type in cases of acute crisis: essential oils of cypress or thyme
- **regulators** of thyroid, endocrine pancreas and adrenal gland function, which, in case of abnormal activity, are always involved in this type of pathology, and are always specific to each patient
- **support** of hepatic and pancreatic function by a diet free of dairy products, animal fats, and foods with a high glycemic index

These various medicinal plants will obviously be chosen according to the condition of the individual child. The use of antibiotics should be reserved for acute infectious episodes affecting those children with an extremely degraded terrain, while the medicinal plants can be maintained as background therapy.

CHAPTER FOUR

Behind the closed doors of the exam room

How I met Dr. Lapraz

I was just getting settled in Paris and was looking for a general practitioner. It was my local pharmacist who first told me about Dr. Lapraz. She was full of enthusiasm because of the highly personalized prescriptions his patients brought in for her to make up. Her recommendation was qualified with: "If you can get an appointment! His office is always packed."

For a few months, I called his number without success, to hear the same message: "Don't call back for at least a month as we are currently not accepting new patients ..." While waiting, I consulted a general practitioner in my neighborhood. He gave me all of ten minutes and seemed bemused by my many various problems. After ordering additional tests, he came up with this wonderful insight: "This is probably the nervous system ... without a doubt it's stress ... perhaps caused by your move?" As for my 4-year-old daughter, who had infectious chickenpox, it was straight onto antibiotics. All done and dusted! I tried to get in a few questions: why antibiotics for chickenpox? Why do I have these shooting chest pains that take my breath away?

These questions seemed to bother him: he was in a hurry all of a sudden, glancing anxiously at his watch. Perhaps he had nothing more to say? Perhaps he was thinking of his dinner or of his waiting room filling up? As he had been tight-lipped and had built his treatment on antibiotics and analgesics, he could claim in all conscience to have done his duty—even though I was left in chronic pain and with daily distress. Knowing that stress was probably the cause of it did not really help!

I continued to call Dr. Lapraz's office without success. In response to my insistent demands, I was told that he keeps late hours and was already struggling to find time for his own patients, to which I continued to reply that I am often ill, with symptoms that are now chronic and are preventing me from leading a normal life.

I did get an appointment in the end, but I had to wait three months! I was told to have blood taken before the appointment and to bring the test results with me.

Three months later, I finally presented myself at his clinic to the surprise of the front desk staff: it seemed that Dr. Lapraz was double-booked! Given it was their mistake, I did not expect to be asked: "Are you sure you have an appointment? You could see another doctor instead: he has trained here and could see you now."

I was not going to be put off: "I have waited three whole months and I want to see this doctor and no-one else."

"Very well, but you will have to wait at least two hours, because he is with a patient at the moment, and it will take a long time."

No problem, I canceled my lunch date and waited ... though I was beset by fears of what might be found out. Like many people, I can be a bit of an ostrich, but there was no point in being faint hearted if this doctor was going to help me get to the bottom of whatever mysteries are going on inside my body. All very worrying! Still, sooner or later, as Bernard Giraudeau says, "we all have to go to the hospital." At least I would hope to be better prepared ...

So, I made up my mind: if this doctor really can come up with a plan of action, I am ready to stay and face the music. If I was going to embrace this holistic approach to the patient, and it might be just what I need, I would have to fight back my fear of what might be uncovered in the process.

Dr. Lapraz came to find me in the waiting room and put his arms around my shoulders in a benevolent manner, as if he had known me for a very long time. Sitting in front of him, in his small office, which was very much in character: austere and unfussy, very much like him, conducive to concentration and trust, I felt immediately at ease.

The time he spent with me gave me permission finally to express what I had been feeling deep down. No other doctor up until then had wanted to listen. Following the thread of our conversation, and taking in his remarks, I began to grasp the coherence and meaning behind my symptoms. Everything was interconnected and hung together, where before nothing seemed to make any sense at all. Our long exchange included an in-depth clinical examination, as no other doctor had done before. It took into account the subtlest sign, relating it with every other sign, to show how over the years I had woven together all my various disorders. Towards the end of the consultation, the assessment of my blood tests provided the physiological explanation for what turned out to be a very good match between my subjective experience and my physical ailments.

In preparation for the appointment, I had brought my blood test results. As well as the usual white and red blood cells, neutrophils, platelets, etc., a few other less standard tests had been requested, such as osteocalcin, a bone protein related to metabolism. All the numbers were within normal range, as they always had been. How was it that nothing showed up, when I felt so awful? For years, I had always been told: "You're in the normal range. There is nothing serious, so don't worry, it is all in your head." And yet, it wasn't *all* in my head …

The consultation: your case could be like mine

Attentive listening

Through his glasses, Dr. Lapraz observed me closely. He asked perceptive, sometimes surprising questions, and often anticipated my replies. This kind of listening was clearly very special. He was interested not only in my lifestyle but in the details of my birth and childhood illnesses, as well as the medical history of my parents and my grandparents. He paid particular attention to seemingly trivial signs: the order in which they appeared, their intensity, relapses, factors which triggered them, and so on. I sensed that all these apparently insignificant details were somehow important. For the first time, I felt someone was listening to me without judgment, and so I felt encouraged to speak without embarrassment or restraint despite my usual shyness.

I began to talk …

I was born in Monaco and my parents worked together in the family business, a pharmaceutical company. As is often the case with couples who work together, they quarreled a lot, often late at night, and this upset me as a child and caused a lot of stress. From a very young age, my mother would confide in me all her doubts and dissatisfactions. I'm sure that my parents loved me but they were hardly ever at home, traveling a lot, and so my childhood wasn't easy. The nannies came and went: it was a lonely childhood.

Towards the end of my adolescence, I had to watch my father begin his long descent into hell. He suffered a stroke with hemiplegia leaving him partly paralyzed. I saw him change from a powerful man into a helpless victim, which affected me very deeply. I admired and loved my father and wanted to care for him, but I felt entirely powerless to deal with his suffering, his pain, and his tears, which I had never seen before. My carefree youth came to an end when faced with the sad plight of my beloved father. After his death, I did not feel that I had the right to live, now that he was gone. I felt guilty for not having been there at his very last moments. In the months that followed I carried on as if nothing had happened, but gradually started to feel depressed as, little by little, I gave myself up to grief.

After I had children, my life took a different perspective and many of the fears and anxieties receded. Many of my physical ailments were diminished or changed. But I am still haunted by an irrational dread of falling ill, triggered by someone I love developing a progressive and incurable degenerative disease. I have a crippling awareness of life's fragility, and this prevents me from ever being truly at ease. Fortunately, I can see my mind at work and at least I know that purposeful activity calms me down. It was at this point that Dr. Lapraz asked me exactly why I had come to see him that day.

"I've had enough of this body which is always giving me trouble!"

It stops me being as active as I'd like and I am brought down by it reminding me, more or less on a daily basis, that all is not well. I try not to think about it and swallow an Acetaminophen (Tylenol®) or a Domperidone to relieve nausea and upset stomach, telling myself it will go away. Since the birth of my second child, 3 years ago, I get colds all the time and suffer with tonsillitis almost continuously. Despite repeated courses of antibiotics, I have chronic ENT inflammation and wake each morning exhausted with a sore throat. Not only the throat, but often with a headache as well, or stomach pain. I also get tingling in my hands and shooting chest pains, close to my heart. These are becoming more frequent, and that worries me.

None of the tests run by my GP (chest X-ray, ECG, endoscopy) has shown up anything abnormal. I've been on antibiotics for long periods for tonsillitis and sinusitis. I've taken an acid blocker (Omeprazole) for months for my stomach problems and anti-inflammatories for migraine headaches. None of these treatments have given me any lasting relief. The worse my symptoms get, the more elusive a cure seems to become. "Dr. Lapraz, are you going to help me understand what is going on in my body? Feeling tired and sick so often is dragging me down. Perhaps you can tell me what it is that I am doing to create all these symptoms? Can you advise me on a healthy diet, attitude and lifestyle that would improve my quality of life?"

Dr. Lapraz seemed to sense in these opening remarks of mine a need for reassurance. It's true that for a long time I had felt the need to talk, to offload a burden that I could not keep putting on those dear to me. I was surprised to find that I was able to talk about things so close to my heart. But this was no casual discussion, and Dr. Lapraz guided our dialog so that I could give him all the details he needed to arrive at his diagnosis. It seems that my answers provided him with all those elements, clearly indispensable, that he needed to come to a definitive assessment of what he called "my terrain."

Attentive listening: identification of my terrain

Everything I said spun an Ariadne's thread which guided the physician through the labyrinth of signs.[1]

A strong emotional reactivity

Dr. Lapraz wanted to know in greater detail about how I experience depression, or how I had reacted to significant events in my life.

I remember that a few months after the death of my father, I was on a plane traveling abroad for my work, and I had an anxiety attack during the flight. I started to feel intense tingling in my hands, my heart was pounding, and panic gripped my throat. I had the impression that nothing and nobody could get me out of this intense heart-rending anxiety. For some time afterwards, I felt that I would never be able to recover, to find inner strength and peace.

The panic attacks carried on for about a year and, strangely enough, tended to come on when traveling in a vehicle, such as car or an airplane, or during certain weather conditions, like unremitting high winds. It was a sensation of an inexorable hurry, the feeling that my life was rushing towards death and that there was nothing I could do to slow it down. Today, these panic attacks are just a bad memory. However, I still feel uneasy when traveling by plane.

Very often, I feel overwhelmed as if my body is trying to tell me something by all these various ailments. For example, I notice that, each year, as fall approaches in September, I am more susceptible to infections, more anxious and irritable, with a drop in energy levels and a low mood.

Cardiac signs that worry me ...

I explained that for a very long time, I have had very troublesome symptoms in the heart area: shooting pains, twitching, spasms, tension, and discomfort in my chest, shortness of breath when walking up a slope, rapid heart rate even at rest, sometimes palpitations. I had all the tests, but the echocardiogram never showed nothing abnormal, and my chest X-ray was completely clear. These symptoms were worrisome particularly as I had a family history of serious heart disease (Osler's disease, an infection that destroys the heart valves causing repeated heart attacks) and yet I was not quite 20 when I first experienced tachycardia, with a heart rate of a 120 beats per minute, though dismissed as not severe by a cardiologist. To regulate my fast and irregular pulse, I had to take a beta blocker, and take regular exercise. I also had poor circulation with cold extremities and my hands would frequently go completely numb.

Recurrent digestive problems ...

I've always had digestive problems. They always start with pain in the pit of my stomach, and I had to have an esophago-gastro-duodenoscopy

(EGD), a test with a barbaric and terrifying name, which involves examining, under light anesthetic, the whole of the stomach up to the duodenum. All it showed was slight inflammation without reflux. I was prescribed a drug (Esomeprazole) designed to reduce stomach acidity, which in my case worked very well, easing the pain very quickly. The trouble is that I have to take it regularly, especially when I get stressed. I can't drink red wine as it immediately gives me heartburn. And I can't drink coffee anymore as I get a reaction in my stomach straight away.

Migraines involving flashing lights

I have suffered from migraine headaches for a long time, particularly with the change of season or work schedule (typically at weekends) and if I drank champagne or white wine. To get rid of them, I would take Doliprane® or Flurbiprofen®, my two wonder drugs!

Dr. Lapraz explained that the weekend migraine is related in part to a change of balance in my autonomic nervous system. As my workload slows down over the weekend, I no longer need to mobilize the part of the system that is involved in movement and activity (the beta-sympathetic), as much as on weekdays when I am much more active. This causes an abrupt change: my parasympathetic, the system of rest and assimilation, takes charge and alters the tone of the cerebral arteries leading to the vasodilation that triggers the migraine attack. By contrast, during the week, my more active beta-sympathetic system curbs this excessive action of the parasympathetic system and so prevents an attack. In addition, we tend to eat more over the weekend which increases demand on the parasympathetic system, which in turn increases the risk of triggering a migraine.

He did not seem baffled or surprised at this long list of disorders and he explained that they are pointers to much older imbalances that he will have to identify.

He pressed me for much greater detail on the emergence and chronology of all my symptoms, as far back as I could remember. He told me that the timeline from birth to the moment they first appeared is essential to enable the physician to establish a coherent medical history. I had to make an effort to remember. Some of these past disorders will be of particular interest to him and allow him to make real progress with his analysis.

Recurrent allergies

During my adolescence, I lived in the South of France and was prone to a lot of allergies. I sneezed a lot, and had red, itchy eyes. I remembered that these allergies had started during a long-haul flight, and stayed with me throughout my adolescence. I had to take Teldane® and Zyrtec® for many years. These allergies disappeared suddenly at about the age of 20, when I moved to Paris and left my childhood home.

Intense dreams, which say a lot about my hormones

Dr. Lapraz asked me to describe my dreams. Their type and content seemed able to provide him with strong clues about how certain hormones were functioning.

I never feel refreshed after a night's sleep with the unpleasant feeling that I have not recovered from the previous day, and yet the sleep studies showed that my sleep is normal. My dreams seem so real that they can wake me up. I remember them throughout the whole of the next day, and their mood persists for a long time. I hardly think of them as dreams; they are more like real life: the sounds and voices, the colors and sensations seemed ever-present along with strong emotions. For example, I could feel a wave of water break over my body, I would cry, or I could experience strong feelings of love or rejection. After these intense nights, I would often wake up tired. In contrast, by the evening and even till late, I would be feeling great.

If a door slams, I am on edge!

I am by nature rather impatient, dynamic, and expressive. I am often in a state of high alert and the slightest emotion can upset me. In general, I tend to be on edge and reactive.

Interpretation: does a hidden thread connect all these signs?

This extensive overview that I've just made of the troubles I am currently experiencing together with those that I have suffered in the past seems so diverse, that I have no idea how Dr. Lapraz can possibly find a connecting thread. Up until now, when consulting a doctor, I would tend to disclose myself piecemeal: my heart to the cardiologist, stomach to the gastroenterologist, migraine headaches to the neurologist, and the troubles of everyday life to my family doctor … And now, after two hours of consultation, everything that bothers me had tumbled out and I had been able to talk about all that has been spoiling my daily life for such a long time.

I was truly perplexed by this mass of signs. I suppose most people are like me, and do not know whom to turn to, once they are told that their condition is not serious …

The beginning of an explanation

Dr. Lapraz told me how to interpret this apparent chaos:

"You know," he told me, "your case is quite normal. Without exception, when we take the time to listen, all patients come out with a huge number of symptoms. Most of these symptoms may seem insignificant, and usually the doctor does not pay too much attention to them. He will be looking out instead for those symptoms that diagnose 'real disease,' those that are recognized by medical science, and which carry a specific label: peptic ulcer, migraine, asthma, or heart attack and so on. By contrast, everything that seems innocuous is considered 'psychosomatic' or is qualified as 'nervousness.' In your case, you were put in the 'anxiety' category since your doctor could not find anything corresponding to a 'real' disease, and therefore, advised you to relax or do more exercise. In other words, such a patient is deemed 'hypochondriac'! However, is it really likely that all these disorders you experience are just the result of random chance? They affect you deeply; otherwise your various doctors would not have put you through all these examinations. Or, rather, can we not find links that may explain why at a certain time your tummy hurts, at another your head makes you suffer or your allergies bother you, or all of these symptoms occur at the same time? Are not all these manifestations a sign of imbalances which need to be identified and corrected as a preventative measure, so that by heeding these alarm bells now we may stop them developing into a far more serious condition? If we neglect these early warnings, future unfavorable events might expose the patient to pathology in the long-term. The problem is that it is not always easy to understand this language of the body. But that should not deter us from trying to find an explanation for the presence of a sign!"

All fired up

Many patients display this intense, edgy personality which correlates with a particular disposition of the nervous system.

"You present, as do so many patients, with a very varied collection of symptoms, which may affect different organs, but which can all be ascribed to the same malfunction of the autonomic nervous system. This system is that part of the nervous system responsible for automatic functioning that lies beyond our voluntary control. It particularly manages the functioning of smooth muscle (digestion and circulation), of cardiac muscle, of most of the exocrine glands (digestion and sweating), and certain endocrine glands (hormones).

Most of your symptoms, and where they show themselves, illustrate quite clearly that your alpha-sympathetic system (a hyper-vigilant stress response) is very strong, and has been for a very long time. This kind of person is easy to spot. Like you, these are people who always display a strong reaction, they are startled when caught off guard, often have digestive spasms and/or repeated migraine headaches, they all have an overactive alert system. This fairly common phenomenon often results from today's lifestyle, which can be very unbalancing (diet and stress, erratic patterns of life with disrupted cycles). That is why so many will recognize themselves in the following symptoms:

The spasmodic state affecting all the organs

This is a mode of nervous system function where the long-term effects of hyper-reactivity will manifest themselves through generalized spasm. These spasms will affect diverse organs and are a testament to a chronic hyper-functioning of the alpha-sympathetic nervous system.

For example, this deep state of hyperactivity may result in an increased production of acid in the stomach. This is why doctors were able to improve your symptoms by prescribing you antacids: they improved your condition at the stomach level, but they did not really heal you. This is only a short-term ploy, an effective one certainly, but still a subterfuge, which will condemn you to dependence on the medication. As the real cause is not located in the stomach but upstream, at the center for autonomic control which is out of kilter, we will not really be able to make this symptom disappear in the long-term, unless we correct the anomaly causing it. If you treat the symptoms of an illness but not its root cause, you should not be surprised by its chronic recurrence.

Migraine headaches are likewise a consequence of a spasmodic state. Here again, in addition to the mechanisms I mentioned with regard to your weekend migraine headaches, medical science tells us that this sign occurs when there is a strong alpha-sympathetic response. And in your case, the risk of migraine is much higher because your body produces *too much histamine*, which is a hormone responsible for the allergies you have had for so long, and which plays an important role in the mechanism of migraine. In addition, one of its effects is to increase the secretion of acid in the stomach!

To complete this explanation about the way your autonomic nervous system works, we need also to talk about the dryness that you very often feel in your throat and which makes you sensitive to the cold. You probably won't be surprised by now to learn that the action of the alpha-sympathetic system on the salivary glands is to dry out their secretion, and therefore dry out the mouth and throat! Another small sign which seems rather unimportant, but which actually tells us a lot!

Similarly, the annoying symptom of cold extremities you feel at bedtime, results also from a temporary alpha-sympathetic hyper-function, because the increase in peripheral capillary tone causes poor circulation. Some people suffer from dead fingers and chilblains in very cold weather: it is a more severe version but poor vasodilation, all the same.

However, that is not all. Other reactions going on in your body confirm, once again, the chronicity of your excessive alpha-sympathetic activity."

Emotional hyper-reactivity

"Is it the case that you are startled when someone pats you on the shoulder or when someone tries to take you by surprise?"

My answer to this question, much as it amuses me, is "yes," and is understood by Dr. Lapraz as a high level of responsiveness and emotionalism, which shows him how my response systems (nervous system, adrenaline discharge, state of the thyroid) function when they are under sudden stress. The nuances in the way the patient expresses his or her reactions (strong startle response or, on the contrary, apathy) will play an important role in the *subtle assessment of the patient's terrain*. For example, there is a huge difference between how a patient suffering from hypothyroidism (where the thyroid is too weak) will react to the same stimulus compared with someone suffering from hyperthyroidism (where the thyroid is too strong). The former subject will remain passive while the latter will be violently startled.

"The reality is even more complex, because a person may have a normal thyroid and still overreact, but for different reasons. The presence of a sign, whether it be obvious or subtle, forms only a part of the overall interpretation. Signs and symptoms have constantly to be re–evaluated before they can be confirmed. In any given case, the doctor must analyze the physiological elements involved and what role they played in the patient. This is because the same sign may have different causes, sometimes acting singly, sometimes in concert. If the thyroid gland seems to be playing a major role, a host of other questions must be addressed to confirm this hypothesis: is the subject thirsty all the time? Does he or she perspire easily? Does he or she have slow tremor at the extremities? If the nervous system is thought to be involved: does the patient have trouble falling asleep or wake up several times during the night? Or complains of early waking? The answers to all these questions enable the physician to identify more accurately the nature of the patient he or she examines.

You suffered repeated stress when you were very young, and your body had to respond. You have modified your response thresholds to these difficulties; thus, you had no choice but to increase your alpha-sympathetic responsiveness, more or less permanently. This has shaped your reaction to aggressions, regardless of their nature. This explains why you sometimes have the impression of overreacting to events or frustrations … This hyper-reactivity plays a considerable part in your various disorders.

Regarding your heart: the shooting pains day and night, the chest discomfort that started several months ago, and the attacks of tachycardia you had when you were only 20. This last symptom alone indicates a particular autonomic balance: not everybody gets tachycardia in their 20s! Yet again, we see evidence of the longstanding hyper-function of your alpha-sympathetic system, an excessive demand which triggers in you a secondary discharge of adrenaline, which in turn is responsible for these attacks of rapid heart rate.

Similarly, the existence of periodic digestive disorders (increased transit, cramps, nausea), occurring during stress, may also be evidence of a discharge of adrenaline as a reaction to the increased activity of the alpha-sympathetic system.

Your bouts of shortness of breath have a particular quality, and are strongly suggestive of a dysfunction of your autonomic nervous system. They occur after the slightest physical effort, or when you walk up the gentlest slope, or increase your pace a little, when climbing stairs, or sometimes even at rest, but often following some emotional upheaval. These symptoms also have a physiological cause and give the doctor clearer ideas towards the most likely diagnosis. These bouts may indicate that your diaphragm has been blocked by alpha-sympathetic stimulation. Such a blockage reduces the capacity of the lungs to adapt to even the smallest demand. Shortness of breath will be the inevitable result from the mismatch between the increased oxygen demand required by the effort and the decrease in the effective volume of air.

At this point in our reflection on the troubles you have shared with me, you will see how the doctor must think when faced with such an array of symptoms. He or she must resort to physiological logic to find coherence in what seems to be incoherent: the diversity of symptoms reported by the patient. It is extremely important to spend time with the patient. As you will have noticed, so far we are only interpreting the signs in their connection with the autonomic nervous system, and even here we have greatly simplified the conclusions we can draw with respect to this system ...

We need to go much deeper now, where the complexity will become even greater.

This is why, to avoid discouraging the reader, we will limit ourselves to the study of some of the disorders you have described:

Our hormones play their part in the background

As much as the autonomic nervous system plays a very important role in the functioning of the human body, it is nevertheless a surface system, so to speak, which is first in line in response to any aggression. A more complex system operates in some ways at a much deeper level, and that is the endocrine system. It ensures the management of the human body at all levels: be it with its structure or with its functionality: the demands placed upon the body in its relationship with the world, its interaction with the external environment. So, the moment you entered my office, smiling, dynamic, excited, quick of speech, and bright of eye, your strong emotional reactivity was immediately obvious, and all this may involve the function of the thyroid gland in a particular way. At first glance, I was given pointers to the particular mode in which your body functions. The information could not have been at all similar if you had a low voice, an inhibited approach, lackluster eyes, or excessive timidity.

The phenomena occurring in the body involves many regulatory systems. That is why the practice of medicine is so difficult, and especially in chronic cases, or in the many pathologies that do not respond to purely symptomatic treatments.

If we confine ourselves to treating symptoms, the appropriate medicinal products act rapidly (for example antibiotics prescribed for acne, or anti-inflammatories for pain) and, given their potency, the symptoms will soon subside. Unfortunately, as soon as the treatment is discontinued, the symptoms reappear, thus condemning the patient to chronicity. Confronted with this limited long-term efficacy of the treatment, the physician should really delve into a deeper understanding of the state of his or her patient. However, contemporary medical training does not prepare doctors to decipher the profound reality hidden behind signs and symptoms. It is the goal of Endobiogeny to propose a more elaborate approach the better to understand the terrain of each individual.

By way of example, you mentioned an interesting detail, namely that before your period, like many women, you felt a pressing need to tidy up. Is there a physiological explanation for this? Thanks to numerous scientific studies, this sign has been found to correlate with a transient increase in the secretion of prolactin, which is the hormone of milk production and growth factors but one that also influences emotional behavior. Prolactin itself is dependent on yet another hormone called thyroid-releasing hormone (TRH). To complicate things further, TRH controls the activity of thyroid hormones. One hormone inside another, rather like Russian dolls. You told me that after you had given birth, you had a lot of milk, so much that it was wouldn't stop flowing in spite of the treatments you were prescribed to stop its production, which is under the control of the prolactin. This demonstrates that you are highly sensitive to this hormone.

All this information provided by patients is what guides us and helps us look behind all the signs, upstream so to speak, so as to understand the complex underlying factors. This way we can get a better understanding of the true state of the patient. Hence, the doctor has to be as careful and precise as possible in the collection of data as patient discusses his or her various ailments. Listening is therefore of the utmost importance.

We are also what we eat

Diet provides important information about the terrain of people who become ill

We went over your dietary habits in some detail as well. This is an important area because of the close links between diet, the digestive tract and the neuroendocrine system. Food, after all, supplies our bodies with the necessary ingredients to function and to feed our cells. There are naturally contrasting needs, of course, between a requirement for instant and intense energy and one that is deep and long lasting. For example, our body needs carbohydrates to be able to respond immediately to the present moment.

It also needs lipids and proteins to ensure the basic maintenance of our structure and to allow it to function properly. Each individual should have a diet according to his or her particular structure, which differs from person to person. Here too, the idea of a diet tailored to each individual, based on his or her terrain, is of great importance and makes you appreciate the potential problems caused when patients succumb to any one of the miracle diets that we are bombarded with. However, what you need to know is that our likes, our dislikes, and our eating habits are not as random as you might think, but closely related to the way in which our hormonal system works. For example, very active and nervous people who burn sugar quickly because of their terrain (with its very active insulin), will tend to prefer cake and bread or drink Coca-Cola, whereas professional athletes who need stamina and muscular strength (which is controlled largely by the adrenal gland) will need protein-rich foods and slow carbs (pasta, rice, pulses).

Taking account of all the details you gave me about your diet provides me with a wealth of information on how your body works in an emergency, and also how it is managed at a deep level.

You told me that you prefer savory to sweet foods. But if I analyze your eating habits carefully, I can see immediately that you eat a large quantity of bread: 2 or 3 slices at breakfast, 4 slices at noon, often

2 to 4 pieces of toast at six in the afternoon if you want a snack, 4 slices in the evening if you eat at home and, as you said, you eat bread while waiting to be served at the restaurant. This adds up to 12 to 15 slices of bread a day, which is a great deal.

What does your appetite for bread mean? It tells us quite simply that you need a lot of energy and without delay because, as we have seen, you use up a great deal of it. Bread, with its very high glycemic index, provides the glucose speedily that your fast metabolism needs. This is why your Biology of Functions finds that you have a high level of insulin activity, which is just what we would expect.

In fact, this hormone is absolutely essential for sugar to enter your cells, which are desperate for it, as they need sugar to function at a high rate. This high level of insulin secreted by your pancreas is, moreover, confirmed by the fact that you get bouts when your energy slumps. There is no question that this results from low blood sugar, because your hyperactive insulin has moved it out of your blood and into your cells so rapidly. This explains your sudden bouts of extreme fatigue: they follow a rapid fall in blood sugar. One further observation that clinches it: your overwhelming urge to sleep right after a meal, which is by no means uncommon, can only be explained by the relationship between insulin and the autonomic nervous system, as those who love an afternoon nap may appreciate. In fact, you use up your insulin— secreted by the pancreas—so quickly that your body has to make some more immediately. To be able to produce it, the pancreas needs to be stimulated by nerves of the parasympathetic system; these not only control the pancreas but also have another major effect in inducing drowsiness. So, you see, the more you need insulin, the more you stimulate your pancreas and inevitably the parasympathetic system as well. As the parasympathetic is in any case fundamental to digestion, your intense fatigue after meals might seem inevitable.

Moreover, this doubtless explains why you cannot tolerate coffee, which, barely ten minutes after drinking it, gives you intense abdominal pain with indigestion. This can be easily be explained by the complex action of coffee: beside its psycho-stimulant action, it can also trigger digestive problems in susceptible patients, like you, because of its effect of raising muscle tone in the digestive tract.

The doctor must pay great attention to the patient's diet, which is where the problem may lie, rather than with the body itself.

So now you begin to grasp how complex the physiological relationships are between the various symptoms a patient may complain of.

Beneath all the multiplicity and diversity, there is an underlying coherence in the deep state (that of the terrain), which unites them. Thus, the heart, the head, the digestive tract, and the airways are each expressing in their own way, a single imbalance.

And one of the great tragedies of modern medicine is that doctors no longer have time to listen to their patients and so come to a full and accurate diagnosis based on a broader approach than just identifying the symptom. There is an urgent need to rethink medical practice entirely; otherwise we run the risk that patients will only be assessed by the modern use of state-of-the-art technologies. No doubt we need these highly advanced machines, but they are not programmed to listen and understand ..."

A crucial step: the detailed examination of the patient's body

The clinical examination, which is a detailed auscultation that follows a precise methodology, is a most important part of the consultation. Just like our discussion prior to the auscultation, this examination will give Dr. Lapraz detailed information about the particular way my body works. "Each sign must be understood in itself, but just as important, in relationship with all the other signs. We then need to reexamine each sign, research and analyze its meaning. This is why the examination of the patient must always be done in a complete and careful manner, with the patient undressed, and not rushed or mechanical, as unfortunately may often be the case these days. And this procedure must not be skipped, even if the doctor has known the patient for a long time: change is part of the dynamic of life and, likewise, symptoms can evolve, both in their appearance, location and intensity, and in their relations with other signs."

A hasty examination can have serious consequences

Failure to discharge this primary responsibility in any medical setting, with all its rigorous demands and procedures, can sometimes have serious consequences for the patient.

"I remember a young man coming into the emergency ward of Boucicault Hospital with a pain in his lower back, which made walking difficult. A month earlier, he had come in with the same symptom and the intern on duty examined his reflexes, which is what you always do when a patient complains of sciatic pain. Not finding any obvious cause, he called the Department head who repeated the examination and briefly checked that the patient was able to stand upright, but still without undressing him. No specific diagnosis was established: The doctor did not come up with a clear diagnosis and dismissed the patient, remarking: 'You probably made an awkward twisting movement. Take this anti-inflammatory and it will soon get better.' But he didn't get any better and the pain persisted.

When he came to see me, the evaluation took a completely different turn, once I took the time to examine him properly. The examination of the undressed patient showed at first glance a serious problem, which had nothing to do with having moved awkwardly! He had on his back a huge malignant melanoma in the lumbar region, which had not been picked up a month earlier. The kind of skin tumor made one suspect that there might well be metastases in the abdomen putting pressure on the sciatic nerve, and so causing pain on walking. This diagnosis was soon confirmed by an emergency scan. Even though a story like this is hardly typical, all too often, unfortunately, patients suffer from clinical examinations conducted with undue haste.

Respect for the system taken as a whole

Once we understand that each sign can be explained not only with the physiology of the organ gives rise to it, but also with other organs and functions of the body, and with the totality of the person, then we realize that we can no longer slice up the sick person into separate and independent pieces. No matter whether the physician is a cardiologist, dermatologist, endocrinologist, gastroenterologist, pulmonologist, gynecologist, immunologist infectious diseases specialist, or psychiatrist, he or she should not be limited to examining the heart, the skin, the endocrine glands, the stomach, the lungs, the breasts, the E. coli or the psyche of the patient being examined, but always consider and examine the patient as a whole.

This integrated global approach ought to be at the heart and soul of all medical practice, and there are plenty of good practical reasons why.

For example, by studying the way your pupils alter when they react to light, as well as how your eyelids respond when my hand approaches your face, and more generally when I check your reflexes, all this tells me about your overall reaction to stimuli. If you blink rapidly when I move my hand quickly towards your forehead, this is a good sign of a strong alpha-sympathetic system. Some patients demonstrate this sign even when they have their eyes closed. The simple fact that they know the hand is going to move close to their face triggers this reflex, even if they do not see the hand and even if the doctor does not move the hand! This shows an extreme vigilance in their alert system ... it is as if they had extra-sensory perception.

As for how your own pupil reacts when a doctor shines a light into your eyes, you can see that this could be taken as an aggression to which your eye has to react, but, you see, the autonomic nervous system is, as its name implies, independent of your will and reacts very quickly, regardless of the organ being examined.

A careful examination of the way the eye responds to light gives the doctor a good deal of information, and I am not talking here about examinations done by the ophthalmologist using high-tech instruments.

Normally the diameter of the pupil decreases when you shine a light beam into it. This constriction of the pupil is called myosis. By contrast, the diameter increases in darkness (mydriasis) to allow more light to enter the eye and reach the retina. These are basic reflexes.

If you look carefully, you will sometimes see people who have widely dilated pupils even in full light. This is a sign of a particular autonomic state: a strong parasympathetic system, with an even stronger response of the alpha-sympathetic. Often, these people are in a state of super-stress or under the influence of drugs. Others, on the contrary, have a very narrow pupil, which is a sign of quite another state of equilibrium.

Watching how the pupil reacts to light is thus very helpful to the doctor in coming to a diagnosis, and it is all very subtle. Indeed, every individual responds differently: one reacts very quickly and his or her pupil becomes very narrow if you keep the light beam on their eye; another will react the same way to begin with, but little by little the pupil's diameter will gradually return to normal; a third, on the contrary, will react very little to the light and his or her pupil will remain very wide; a fourth will present rapid alternations of constricted and dilated pupils (the so-called pupillary pulse).

All the information gained will be crucial in choosing the treatment best suited to the patient.

In this broader vision, a more comprehensive approach is taken to all these signs, seen in all their subtlety. They give me a very clear idea about your high level of reactivity by which I mean your sympathetic nervous system that I have been watching since we started our discussion, especially with respect to a substance with a marked influence on the brain and behavior, and that is *dopamine*. As an indicator, the way in which the lower eyelid reacts when I tap the forehead with my finger gives an idea of how this neurotransmitter is operating.

This substance plays a role in several vital functions: mood, sleep, behavior, the ability to learn, attentiveness, and motor skills. Now, the stresses you suffered since you were very young has led to an excessive activation of your dopamine, which, in turn, has activated your adrenaline and, therefore, your general reactivity. This may also explain, at least in part, the restlessness in your legs, your rapid heart rate, your light and disturbed sleep, your intense dreams ...

As we continue your clinical examination, the distribution of your body fat, the size and shape of your fingers, and of your face, the brightness of your eyes, your tone of voice, your flow of speech, the muscle tone of your abdomen, the presence of spots in certain parts of your body, the color of your tongue (and whether it has cracks in the middle, the shape of your palate, all these signs, and so much more, that most physicians don't take the time to look for and analyze, are all incontrovertibly important if we want to understand exactly how you are made and how you function."

Dopamine deficit or excess: two types of personalities

The signs presented by those in whom dopamine production and activity are abnormal are an important indicator of how their psyche functions.

The very annoying disorder of *restless leg syndrome*, which usually comes on in the evening or at bedtime, can often be due to increased dopamine—despite what current research indicates. What is key is to understand that the master thyroid hormone, TRH, is also elevated and plays a role with dopamine. If you feel anxious during the day, are easily startled or have intense or vivid dreams, this may be the case with you. This leads to a vicious circle: in a state of excessive nervous tension, the secretion of dopamine tends to rise further and sleep, which is under the control of serotonin (a hormone, which is also closely connected with depression), may be disturbed because of this imbalance between dopamine and serotonin: restful sleep becomes elusive. This sleep disturbance compounds the problem and the person wakes feeling exhausted.

1—Those with dopamine deficiency:

These individuals are recognized by their tendency to depression and lack of energy, their emotional withdrawal and inhibited disposition or even autistic tendencies, with poor psychomotor coordination (dyspraxia) and cognitive disorders.

An extreme deficiency of dopamine may lead eventually to Parkinson's disease. Recent studies have shown that estrogen plays a major role in maintaining dopamine levels: a lack of estrogen may result in a 30% decline in cerebral dopamine and may dispose to the development of Parkinson's disease.

2—Those with dopamine excess:

These are often people who are extremely anxious and very excitable, who display hyper-vigilance and are very emotional, often with a rapid heart rate or high blood pressure. In extreme cases, they may be prone to hallucinations, and may lead them on to mania or paranoid psychosis with illusions and delusions.

Another decisive step: the analysis of the indexes in the biology of functions

"The individual and his or her terrain revealed in a drop of blood."

This last step will complete the clinical picture of the patient. In cases where it is applicable, the doctor will at this point analyze and integrate all the data gathered from other investigations such as scans of all sorts, X-rays and mammography, and the findings from the testing of various bodily samples.

The Biology of Functions, depending on the values of each of the indexes obtained from the blood test, will either confirm or call into question the conclusions reached in the previous steps of the consultation and the physical examination.

Indexes That Speak

These numerical values, called "indexes," are derived a sample of blood taken in the usual clinical way. To the results obtained from these standard blood tests, algorithms are applied that are based upon scientific data already published in the scientific literature or on recognized norms. They reveal a hidden truth, much more detailed and more than you get by looking at each of the standard results in isolation. They allow us to quantify, and therefore identify objectively, the subtle connections between the organs and the various functions of the human body. They give the doctor a much more detailed overview of the real state of the patient, and so help direct him or her to a much more effective treatment plan or preventative strategy. They are based on the proposition that it is our hormonal system that orchestrates and manages all of life's mechanisms, that it controls from moment to moment the functioning of our whole organism at every level, from molecular and cellular, to the tissues and organs. One of the great strengths of these indexes, and a fundamental concept, allows for them to be continuously validated and updated even on a daily basis. (see Chapter 3: A True Terrain-Based Medicine: A New Hope for Patients, the paragraph entitled "The Biology of Functions" on p. **).

What do these values say about my hormones?

In my case, these indexes indicate that the overall activity of my ovaries is rather low, and the pituitary gland is overactive in trying to upregulate their function. Dr. Lapraz tells me that this biological sign is often found in women in their 40s and reflects a transitional hormonal imbalance that may last for about a year. In fact, it is quite common for them to complain to their gynecologist of irritability, night sweats and dry skin. In other words, similar troubles to those that occur much later, at the menopause, and which reflect a more prolonged imbalance between estrogen, progesterone, and the pituitary gland. It is as if all women between the ages of 38 and 42 stage a rehearsal of the menopause, which is expected to arrive a decade later.

This puts me in mind of my friend Claudia, a very beautiful 40-year-old woman, telling me that she feels a change in her body (dry skin, night sweats, unexplained nervousness) and doesn't know what to put it down to. Her gynecologist reassured her that her blood tests results showed no hormonal abnormality, and as everything was normal she has no reason to worry.

Dr. Lapraz explained that there is a discrepancy between the symptoms experienced by these women and the apparent normality of the blood test results. In fact, it is possible for there to be a real estrogen deficiency in the body at tissue level, which gives rise to the symptoms, while the level of estrogen as measured in the blood is normal or even high. This paradox can be explained by the integrative approach taken by the Biology of Functions, which is able to identify the actual estrogen activity at tissue level.

With regard to my *thyroid*, it is the analysis of the results provided by a set of indexes, each one assessing the specific action of this gland on the whole body,[2] that will allow Dr. Lapraz to establish a deeper, more comprehensive understanding of the role it actually plays in my disorders. The set of indexes shows that the activity of my thyroid is significantly raised (but not to a dangerous level), and thus confirms the assessment he made from his clinical examination.

This supports my account of animated dreams—because the thyroid plays the role of artistic director of our dreams—and, more generally, it can be seen in my keen and lively demeanor. "This is the case with many of my patients," Dr. Lapraz confides, "but we can go much further in assessing the role played by this gland in the origin and development of a variety of conditions. The analysis of particular indexes, such as, for example, those that assess the status of thyroid activity at the change of seasons, allows us to understand the acute relapses of certain serious diseases during these times of the year, corroborated by clinical studies carried by American colleagues."[3]

Another significant finding is that the insulin activity in my body is three times higher than normal. The role of insulin is to transfer glucose out of the blood and into the cells and so a large quantity of this fundamental fuel gets into mine. This is hardly surprising, given my frequent overstressed state, as stress consumes a huge amount of energy. As with so many people today, this extreme cellular activity is caused by having to cope with the demands of modern life and the time pressure it imposes. Excessive cellular activity is inevitably associated with a high level of oxidation, and will in my case require the prescription of antioxidants. In fact, my body produces a great number of free radicals, and these behave very aggressively toward my cells and tissues. Contrary to current popular opinion, which advises everyone to take antioxidants, Dr. Lapraz maintains that balancing redox reactions is a highly complex adaptive mechanism, and so it can be hazardous to take antioxidants without due cause. "A prescription is ill-suited to a patient who presents with a deficiency rather than an excess of oxidation and may well prove detrimental. There is a great risk of causing oxidation deficiency in such a patient, and over the medium- or long-term, this may lead to degenerative diseases, such as Alzheimer's or cancer."

My allergy markers show that I have a very high *histamine index*, and reflects biologically the allergic susceptibility of the mucous membranes of my nasal passages. When my blood was taken, the test protocol did not actually request levels of histamine to be measured and reported, but the Biology of Functions allows us to assess its activity at the tissue level.

In fact, histamine plays a crucial role in this type of hypersensitivity of the throat and airways, and may explain why I am so prone to repeated colds and sore throats, especially when exposed to air conditioning.

The doctor as detective

When these explanations drew to a close, I began to appreciate why Dr. Lapraz took so much time to listen to me. He needed to collate all the symptoms I reported with the signs he elicited so that he could begin to understand the state of my terrain.

"Nothing happens in the body just by chance. Just as warning lights flicker on and off at different times, so *all* symptoms must all be taken into account and pieced together, irrespective of whether someone comes with simple and common symptoms, or is a patient who presents during an advanced stage of a disease. With follow-up appointments, my job is to identify any changes in the expression of my patients' symptoms, however innocuous they might seem; this allows me to adjust my therapeutic choices in keeping with the evolution of the terrain. This way I can provide truly preventative and supportive medical care."

There is an impressive logic at work behind these links that Dr. Lapraz makes. As all parts within an individual are inseparably bound together, one can see that by listening to a patient's complaints, and analyzing the clinical and biological signs, everything fits together and each sign brings its share of vital information. It would make no sense, then, to formulate a treatment plan that limited itself merely to treating symptoms. In my case, I was given a preventative treatment aimed at correcting those imbalances in which I was embroiled. It was a personalized prescription, designed for maximum efficacy and minimum toxicity. It was adapted to my needs and supported my weak points: it aimed not only to rebalance my terrain but also to prevent any deterioration of my condition. Otherwise, I might sooner or later go further down the road into ill–health and develop some serious pathology.

*The last step of the consultation: the least toxic possible treatment
for long-term effectiveness*

A conventional treatment?

"Any general practitioner is bound to prescribe formulaic treatments
for each condition, as is defined by the consensus of medical opinion
and the Ministry of Health.

Based on the diagnosis of quite a few of your disorders affecting
several of your organs, I could reasonably prescribe for you the following, according to the conventional medical approach:

- a beta blocker, to regulate your rapid heart rate,
- an anti-inflammatory, to relieve your migraine headaches,
- an antihistamine, to treat the allergic component of your repeated
  colds,
- a medicinal product to reduce the amount of gastric acid produced
  by your stomach (proton pump inhibitors (PPIs),
- an antispasmodic, to calm your digestive pain and spasms,
- progesterone, to boost and normalize your ovarian function."

Benefits

"The apparent benefits of taking these medicinal products are obvious:
speedy and effective action in the short-term with immediate relief
from the symptoms. The stomach pain disappears as if by magic, the
heart slows down soon after the first tablet is taken, anxiety dies down
within minutes, the migraine is likewise gone, and your menstrual
cycle will be regulated ... But, Marie-Laure, you have already taken all
these treatments a number of times, and yet they have failed to change
your underlying state because as soon as you stop taking them, your
troubles by and large return, quite unchanged, to haunt and disturb
you. Doesn't this lead you to ask yourself whether you might have a
serious disease that the doctors have missed?"

Disadvantages

"Aside from that possibility, the other disadvantage to the instant relief
promised by these medicines concerns their many possible adverse
effects. These are by no means negligible and their toxicity is well

known (think of the case of Celebrex mentioned on page 38), and so may contribute to non-compliance by the more sensitive patient.

Furthermore, in cases where these drugs are prescribed inappropriately the harm they do is in proportion to the pharmacological power they exert on the body. In addition to these well-documented side effects, these medicinal products may give rise to other undesirable outcomes. These may be less obvious and more subtle, but not less damaging than those of direct toxicity because of their potential to unleash a cascade of influences upon other systems of the human body, especially when they are taken over a long period of time.

These medicines taken for short periods from and time to time don't really cause a lot of harm. However, their abusive and widespread use is a real social problem that medicine is powerless to control.

Another drawback: if powerful medication is given in order to replace the function of a failing organ, the organ in question will not recover function as long as the treatment continues and will delay or prevent the body's ability to regulate itself, making it even more dependent on the prescribed product. For example, taking a synthetic progestin will provide immediate benefit, but in the long-term, it will reduce the ovary's ability to make its own progesterone.

While it may be acknowledged that these synthetic medical compounds need to be prescribed in exceptional cases, for the majority of patients a less toxic and more personalized therapeutic choice is to be preferred, at least in the first instance, with highly potent products reserved as a treatment of last resort.

In my 40 years in daily general practice, I have come to the conclusion that most patients, currently on synthetic drugs, would do very well on treatments that are less harmful to their body and better adapted to its physiology; these would not only improve their present condition but would in the long run heal them. Unfortunately, therapeutic choice that is less harmful for the patient has been deliberately swept aside in France and is not recognized as approved medical practice by the Social Security authorities."

Is there another way: a natural, less toxic plant-based treatment?

What overall outcome can be expected?

"Any treatment strategy (after considering the patient's need for immediate relief) must be founded on a plan that ensures the various underlying dysfunctions are corrected. As with every patient, these were identified through your history and clinical examination, as well as by the results from your Biology of Functions. These provide the medical practitioner with a tool to bring focus to the choice of therapeutics but is entirely dependent, once again, of taking a holistic approach that includes all available data.

When deliberating on the choice of your initial treatment, we must first define our objectives and place the changes we want to bring about in order of priority. The theme that emerges most clearly is your excessive alpha-sympathetic reactivity. This kind of excess activity will burden several organs so it is essential to support their functioning, especially your digestive tract, bearing in mind that your pancreas has been put under great stress by the chronically raised insulin activity. Even so, your condition does not actually call for harsh and potent treatment, so we will set up a course of Phytotherapy for you and solely use medicinal plants, choosing those that are supported by scientific studies published internationally in English.[4]

A good number of medicinal plants could qualify for inclusion in your treatment, but we must be selective. We'll choose those that work synergistically or facilitate the desired physiological effects, or provide the benefit of drainage. We often need to call upon this action when patients have taken medicinal products for years, as you have done, and these have overloaded the organs. Drainage by plants will help with cleansing and detoxification, especially the liver and intestines.

Some will even reduce the excessive activity in your alpha-sympathetic system, notably essential oils of lavender and petit grain, and whole-plant extracts of hawthorn. These plants are endowed with significant sedative effects on the central nervous system, and they can also exert a positive influence on cardiac hyper-excitability, and so reduce the likelihood of tachycardia. The great advantage of choosing them is that they we can also benefit from their appreciable antispasmodic action on the digestive system, which as we know is one of the areas in which you are most affected.

Whole-plant extracts of walnut, plantain, and rosemary may also contribute to your ability to absorb nutrients. They do so by their specific actions on the liver (drainage) and pancreas (support and regulation of insulin activity). They also have astringent, anti-inflammatory and anti-gastritis activity, and these complementary and synergistic actions will reduce the tendency of your tissues towards inflammation.

Some of the plants chosen have antihistamine and anti-allergic properties as well (agrimony, blackcurrant, plantain) while others reduce microbial activity in the respiratory passages (cinnamon, lavender, blackberry) and so tend to reduce the hypersensitivity of your nasopharyngeal mucosa.

Finally, others such as the yarrow, lady's mantle, alfalfa, and sage can bring much-needed estrogenic and progestogenic support to your ovary during this phase of hormonal imbalance you are currently experiencing.

Given that we use very low doses—more than a thousand times lower than those of synthetic drugs—we need to choose very carefully plants that are synergistic or complementary to ensure a really beneficial outcome.

Each plant, by contributing small effects in a collective way, leads to an overall improvement and then may lead to a lasting cure. Because of the low doses we use, this additive process reduces the risk of unwanted effects that any one of them might cause if they were taken in a much higher dose.

You are thus treated at several levels all at the same time thanks to the multiplicity of effects that each of the chosen plants brings to bear upon your overall condition.

Fundamental laboratory research or animal studies and research from clinical practice have clearly demonstrated that lavender essential oil has the following actions: analgesic, anti-myalgic, anti-neuralgic, pelvic decongestant (through venous stimulation), anti-inflammatory and anti-allergic, choleretic, anticoagulant, (by opposing vitamin K), hypotensive. It has anti-microbial properties (particularly against streptococcus and staphylococcus) on the skin, and in the respiratory and genitourinary systems as well as in the bile ducts and the intestinal tract generally. It is also diuretic and antispasmodic to the urinary passages, and above all is sedative due to its ability to reduce tone very effectively in both the alpha-sympathetic and parasympathetic systems.

This plant is an obvious choice for you: while lowering both your overall hyper-excitability and the threshold at which you react, it will also lower your tendency to uterine cramp reduce the likelihood of urinary and respiratory infections, dampen the allergic response, and lower the tone in capillary vessels.

I chose it for these reasons, and in your particular case, for its benefits to the circulation and its sedative and analgesic effect on the nervous system, as well as for its antispasmodic, anti-allergic, anti-inflammatory, and anti-infective properties. The combination of all these effects means that it can be just as valuable in patients who present with a very different symptom picture: it is the imbalance that lurks behind their disorder for which we seek all these diverse therapeutic actions. One needs always to take care that by using a plant to assuage a patient's symptoms, you do not end up exacerbating deeper terrain imbalances, and thus defeat the object of this more comprehensive approach.

For example, it would not make sense to include in your prescription a plant that would oppose the action of lavender by increasing the tone of your alpha-sympathetic system.

This treatment aims to utilize your body's innate capacity for self-healing. By prescribing natural products with clearly defined physiological effects in low doses we aim to help you achieve a better state of overall balance with the least toxicity. As an additional benefit, your reliance on synthetic drugs will usually be greatly reduced. These powerful substances that you have been prescribed up until now take over the functions of your own body and do nothing to induce self-healing."

I returned home armed with my prescription and with my head buzzing after this visit. This was the first time that I had been able to understand how my body functions and how everything was interconnected and the deep reasons behind the treatment that I had been prescribed.

Perhaps you would also like to try and identify the strengths and weaknesses of your own terrain?

CHAPTER FIVE

What type of terrain are you?

A re we all equal when faced with disease? Or are there differences from birth in our ability to maintain ourselves in good health? Reality tends to show that equality does not exist: why does one two-month-old infant develop acute weeping eczema, while another infant in the same crèche has perfect skin? Why does one have five ear infections over the winter and fails to thrive, while the baby next-door flourishes?

Once it is understood that the type of each individual's terrain predicts the most likely course taken by their maladies, it is reasonable to address the issue of terrain from earliest childhood. Indeed, each of us comes into the world with our own terrain. Using the analogy of types of car, you could say that each terrain ranges from a Citroen 2CV to a Ferrari, but this says very little and tells us nothing about how well or badly one functions compared to another.

Generally speaking, we encounter two major types of people:

- Those with moderate imbalances in the baseline terrain and generally enjoying good health with occasional minor reactions to any
disturbances. They do not present with unusual or particular sets of
symptoms.

- Those whose symptoms reflect their underlying fragility and for whom preventative care from a very early age would confer great benefit. The majority of people fall into this category and may often feel unwell. Their overall equilibrium is more or less fragile. They tend to exhibit a great variety of symptoms, which are indicators of a weakness in an organ, a function, or a system. These signs and symptoms appear in all shapes and sizes: debility, anxiety, palpitations, a perennial sensation of a lump in the throat, dizziness, nausea, insomnia, depression, muscle pain, digestive spasms, colitis, constipation, diarrhea, cystitis, menstrual disorders, frigidity, or impotence, and the list goes on … They reflect the existence of an abnormality that, if neglected, can lead to more serious illness. This language of the body always has a meaning and is the culmination of intense and profound imbalances (either few or many) that grow and develop over the years. The earlier these symptoms show up the more they testify to the fragility of the underlying structure of that person.

These maladies are usually chronic or recurrent. They greatly reduce the quality of life and may incapacitate the sufferer and provide the physician with his daily bread. These conditions tend to get worse over time and may eventually turn into an intractable disease. Whether that happens will depend upon the type and severity of the initial imbalance in the terrain, but also, of course, on how challenging and stressful life has been and how severe, lasting, and repeated major traumas were and, crucially, how the terrain of that person responded.

Can one get some idea about a person's terrain?

An Endobiogenic assessment enables the doctor to evaluate the patient's terrain with great accuracy.

As each human being is unique[1] and so cannot really be assigned to a category, it might seem something of a contradiction to attempt to define the major types of terrain. However, it is possible to correlate gross morphology and personality traits with a certain type of terrain just as we can relate clinical signs with a predisposition to certain diseases and even their progression, but none of these observations amount to a system of pigeonholing people.

Both the autonomic nervous system and the endocrine system are involved in the structure and management of the terrain. The autonomic nervous system is in charge of our adaptive response from moment to moment while the endocrine system exerts deeper more lasting control.

The autonomic nervous system, your unseen worker

Before presenting in table form those characteristics that will give readers a chance to work out their terrain for themselves, we should first take a moment to recall how the ever-present autonomic nervous system works for us.

The regulation of digestion as an example of the autonomic system

Our digestion is a complex phenomenon that depends upon the coordination of several mechanisms. Food has to be propelled the whole length of the digestive tube in coordination with secretions of a variety of juices and enzymes that break down what we have eaten so as to release the nutrients and then assimilate them. This timing of these secretions from the liver and pancreas, with the transport of food along the entire length of the digestive tract, from the mouth to the anus, is critical for good digestion. These motor and secretory phenomena have to operate in tandem in a harmonious manner and in a specific order.

All these phenomena at the digestive tract level are coordinated and regulated by the nervous system, and is beyond our control, as the name "autonomic" suggests.

The autonomic nervous system operates automatically and in three parts or phases, each playing a different and complementary role to the other two. If one of them is faulty, either by excess or deficiency, or if it acts too soon or too late, we can expect to suffer any number of digestive disorders.

- The parasympathetic system (under the influence of the neurotransmitter acetylcholine) regulates the basal muscle tone of the walls and therefore the propulsion of food along the digestive tract and, at the same time, stimulates the digestive secretions and initiates digestion.

- The alpha-sympathetic system (under the influence of noradrenaline) sets the controls of the sphincters that line the digestive tract. Sphincters are tiny circular bands of muscle that act like gates: they open or close in anticipation of a meal or in response to its arrival, and thereby dictate how long or short a time food remains in contact with the digestive enzymes, and so they have the potential for slowing intestinal transit. Very sensitive to stress, sphincters can easily go into spasm, causing stomach pain and poor digestion.
- The beta-sympathetic (under the influence of adrenaline) works in conjunction with the tone initiated by the parasympathetic and responds to the bulk of food being digested: by relaxing the initial high tone further down the gut, it ensures the effective transit of food along the whole tract. Thus, the parasympathetic initiates, the alpha-sympathetic regulates and the beta-sympathetic opens the tract to allow the completion of the digestive process with the evacuation of undigested matter.

You can appreciate how easy it would be for such a delicate mechanism to get out of sync and cause a lot of trouble. If the secretions are too abundant from excessive parasympathetic activity or excessive discharge of adrenaline, abdominal bloating and distention will occur, with diarrhea. If, on the other hand, we struggle with chronic stress, that puts us into a state of permanently raised alpha-sympathetic tone. This state of chronic tension in the muscles that coat the digestive tract tends to lead to chronic constipation. However, things get more complicated because these three systems always follow one another in this sequence:

First, the parasympathetic,
Then, the alpha-sympathetic, and
Lastly, the beta-sympathetic and then the cycle starts again.

If, for example, the parasympathetic system drives too strongly, the other two systems will react immediately. The quality of this reaction will differ from person to person because the capacity of our alpha and beta systems to adapt to change is highly individual. As these three parts of the autonomic nervous system operate throughout the body, we shouldn't confine ourselves to studying the digestive tract if we want to try and figure out what else is going on in the body of our patient; we need to look elsewhere for other signs to support our diagnosis.

Why look elsewhere? Because the functioning of the digestive tract does not depend solely on the autonomic nervous system, but also on the hormonal balance and on every aspect of the person as a whole. Only by addressing ourselves to this great complexity can we hope to understand the real state of each individual.

What kind of terrain do you have?

The tables[2] below give an account of the activity of the autonomic nervous system on the body as a whole and should be read as follows:

- Each branch of the autonomic nervous system has been shown separately to illustrate how each of them affects the body, either in attitude and behavior or by the signs each tends to induce and the attendant risks for that person, depending on whether they tend to hyper-function or hypo-function);
- The more a person exhibits "hyper" or "hypo" signs, the more likely they are to be under the dominance of the relevant autonomic category.

For example, if you are rather timid, if your heartbeat is slow and your blood pressure low, with warm and moist extremities, and are subject to bloating and flatulence and you are prone to recurrent bouts of bronchitis, then your terrain may be under the dominant influence of the parasympathetic system.

On the other hand, if you are frequently irritable with a quick temper, experience hot flashes and have a rapid pulse with a tendency to hypertension and diabetes, then you are probably on the far side of a dominant beta-sympathetic system.

Conversely, if you are permanently tired and exhausted by the slightest effort, suffer from asthma or have a tendency to sudden herpes outbreaks, all these symptoms indicate an insufficiency of the beta-sympathetic system.

Of course, there may be other explanations for all these dispositions, hormonal ones in particular, as we will see later. However, the tables below will give you some idea of how your autonomic system works.

	Strong parasympathetic	Strong alpha-sympathetic	Strong beta-sympathetic
Your behavioral tendencies	Timid, introverted, anxious, shy with a tendency to inhibition, uncomfortable with public speaking. The parasympathetic is a system of rest, assimilation, and recovery.	Hypersensitive, with a heightened esthetic sense, intolerance to noise and other stimuli with all senses highly tuned, hypersensitivity to pain, and to cold. In a state of permanent tension, and anxious arousal. The alpha-sympathetic system is the system of vigilance.	An impulsive, agitated person, fidgety and restless, unable to stand still, irritable, prone to violent outbursts of anger, expansive but with a tendency to aggression, prone to panic attacks. The beta-sympathetic system is a fighting and movement system, which responds to mental or physical stimulation.
Signs	Rather flat thorax, often with sternum somewhat sunken, face rather rounded with thin hair, limbs warm and sweaty, pupils constricted (myosis) with a tendency to long-sightedness, low blood pressure with a slow, full pulse, subject to extrasystoles, inspiratory time longer than	Tendency to myopia, dilated pupils (mydriasis), cold, or very cold hands and feet, cold knees, varicosities in a pale palate, red (but cold) face, red ears and cheekbones, cold sweat in the armpits, palms of hands, and soles of feet, skin responds to friction with red patches (dermographism), rapid movement of the upper eyelid, tongue exhibits fine tremor,	Bounding pulse, rapid heart rate, frequent palpitations, tremor of the hands which are dry and warm, hot flashes, alternates between pale and flushed and face with red cheekbones, wavering voice, rate and volume of pulse increases when undergoing a medical examination.

	expiratory time, abundant watery secretions from the linings of nose, throat and sinus, and in the chest and along the digestive tract, with copious saliva.	expiratory time shorter than inspiratory time, dry mouth and mucous membranes, with tongue sticking to roof of mouth, systolic murmur heard on auscultation of the abdomen.	Diarrhea, vomiting, hypertension, diabetes.
Problems	Generalized sweating, sweating in the early part of the night, flatulence, abdominal bloating, pelvic congestion, tendency to develop varicose veins, bronchitis, gastritis, colitis with diarrhea, psoriasis, eczema; in extremis, vagal crisis: dizziness, nausea, sweating, vomiting.	Tendency to spastic constipation from hypertonic intestinal smooth muscle, subject to vomiting, insomnia, irritability, tendency to streptococcal infection, herpes, psoriasis, eczema, and conditions with a strong spasmodic component: migraine, asthma, peptic ulcer, etc.	

	Weak parasympathetic	Weak alpha-sympathetic	Weak beta-sympathetic
Your behavioral tendencies	Hypercritical of self or passive-aggressive combined with a sluggish or lethargic temperament.	Major adaptation difficulties.	The slightest effort seems to be a mountain, lack of cravings and desires, constant fatigue blocking any initiative, absence of libido.
Signs	General deficiency: weak heart rate, weakness of cardiac contractions, very low diastolic pressure (the bottom number) (120/60, for example), little developed musculature, muscle weakness, cold and dry extremities, tendency to mydriasis, hands rather cold and dry.	The passage from parasympathetic to beta-sympathetic is not correctly done, therefore, there will be either signs of strong parasympathetic (see above), or signs of weak beta-sympathetic (see right hand column), tendency to myosis.	Chronic and constant fatigue, the batteries are flat, hands rather warm, normal heartbeat but with hypotension, the diastolic (bottom number) is balanced in relation with the systolic pressure (top number) (110/70, for example), hypohidrosis (lack of sweating).
Problems	Constipation caused by scanty intestinal secretions; nightmares, hallucinations.	See: disorders under strong parasympathetic and weak beta-sympathetic; veins are often dilated.	Waking dreams, split personality, cerebral and coronary arterial and cerebral circulatory insufficiency due to a lack of adrenaline, which normally acts to dilate the arteries carrying blood to vital organs; risk of respiratory disease from poor bronchial dilatation (asthma), tendency to allergies, migraines, and severe outbreaks of herpes.

Let us now turn to those characteristics that may be related to an overall reduction of activity in the autonomic nervous whether it is found in the parasympathetic or alpha-sympathetic or beta-sympathetic systems.

Which hormone do you rely on the most?

We have seen that the endocrine system is the manager of our body's structure and is responsible for the way we adapt in response to any stressful challenge.

It is possible, then, for everyone to get some idea of how their body functions by carefully examining a range of possible symptoms.

The following table lists the signs and the symptomatic tendencies attributable to some of the hormones that we mapped in the diagram of the four endocrine axes presented in Chapter 3: corticotropic, gonadotropic, thyrotropic, and somatotropic.

If we take ACTH first (standing for Adreno-Corticotropic-Hormone and so belongs in the corticotropic axis): this is secreted in response to stress and triggers our adaptation system. This provides us immediately with the energy we need. One can get an idea of how active ACTH is in our body by checking for certain signs:

	Strong ACTH	Weak ACTH
Your behavioral tendencies	Tendency to extroversion, bad memory.	Adaptation difficulties, tendency to severe depression.
Signs	Accumulations of fat on the upper part of the back (buffalo hump), hairs in the ears, hyperpigmentation, oral mucosa with hyper-pigmented spots, tendency to increased blood sodium.	Intense asthenia, depigmentation (particularly breast areolae and genital organs). See also signs of low cortisol.

(*Continued*)

	Strong ACTH	*Weak ACTH*
Problems	Early morning waking, pruritus on the thighs, congestion in the pit of the stomach, palpitations, acne on the back, pronounced stretch marks, particularly on the inner thighs and the trunk; eczema, psoriasis, endocrine disorders with high cortisol levels.	Hypoglycemia, tendency to hypotension.

Thus, if you are a rather extroverted individual, wake up early in the morning, have a good short-term memory, and you have pronounced stretch marks on your thighs, a pad of fat on your upper back (the "buffalo hump," as it is known), and if you also get palpitations, eczema, or psoriasis, then, it is quite likely that your ACTH activity is too high, either permanently or quite frequently.

Cortisol levels may also be evaluated through the careful study of certain signs. Cortisol is a hormone secreted by the adrenal gland and plays a crucial role in all the biochemical reactions that occur in the body (metabolism of sugars, fats, protein, as well as water, and mineral balance). Most importantly, it enables all the other endocrine glands to function properly.

However, when a person is put under major stress, their body secretes large quantities of cortisol, so-called adaptive cortisol, which puts a block on the body's normal functioning for the duration of the emergency. The extent of this blockage and how long it lasts depends, of course, on the nature of the stress, but the more intense and the longer it lasts, the more damaging will be the effects. The situation needs to be corrected at all costs to avoid the development of serious disease.

This is why it is so important to reduce long-term emotional stress by any practice that utilizes our own abilities to restore inner harmony;

there is an enormous amount of medical research and an extensive literature on the subject with a huge range of books on the subject. One example among many is by David Servan-Schreiber.[3]

	Strong cortisol	Weak cortisol
Your behavioral tendencies	Chronic stress, depression, hyper-reactivity.	Lack of responsiveness.
Signs	Cellulite on the inner arms and thighs with muscle wasting, excess belly fat, excessive fat around neck and supraclavicular fossae, delicate and fragile skin and capillaries, tendency to bruise and form little red spots on the skin, purple stretch marks on the hips, abdomen, and breasts.	Asthenia, fatigability, hypotension, tendency to being thin, delayed puberty.
Problems	Overweight, accumulation of fat in the tissues, osteoporosis with back pain, risk of fracture, cessation of menstruation, chronic infections, and tendency to depression, fungal infections, diabetes, hypertension, raised blood lipids, Cushing disease (excess cortisol from the adrenal gland or from medication with cortisone).	Chronic fatigue, hoarseness, susceptibility to infections, acne, asthma, eczema, herpes, psoriasis.

So, if you have large patches of cellulite on your arms and thighs, with pigmented stretch marks on your trunk or breasts, or you have a lot of thread veins, and if you have a tendency to depression and catch a lot of colds or other infections, and have high blood pressure, then it is more than likely that your cortisol level is too high. But here again, we cannot be too dogmatic in our interpretation; we have to take all these signs together with other signs induced by other hormones that can interfere on these same signs and have effects that are more or less similar.

These first two hormones that we have just studied, ACTH and cortisol, belong to the corticotropic axis, and as the axis of rapid mobilization of energy is the first line of response to any aggression.

Let us look now at those hormones involved in the second phase of adaptation, the *gonadotropic axis*. This *renewal* phase is charged with the provision of materials, mostly in the shape of structural proteins and enzymes, that allow the body to build and repair itself and maintain normal function.

The secretion of follicle stimulating hormone (FSH) from the pituitary gland initiates this axis. We can get an idea of the strength of its secretion in a person by how they tend to behave as well as the presence or absence of certain signs in their bodies.

	Strong FSH	*Weak FSH*
Your behavioral tendencies	Highly sensitive, strong femininity.	Weak or absent libido.
Signs	Cellulitis on inner parts of upper legs and arms, more pronounced on the right than the left; fine hair and long eyelashes; pigmented spots on elbows and knees; redness of the smile creases, violet-colored tonsils.	Amenorrhea in girls, pubertal delay, and deficient development of secondary sexual characteristics in both sexes; small breasts, small penis; difficulty in gaining weight.
Problems	Sensitivity of the ascending (right) colon, presence of hard and more or less tender areas in the breast, mainly on the right; psoriasis, acne, eczema; Crohn's and other inflammatory bowel diseases especially in the right colon.	Decreased libido, erectile dysfunction. Loss of menstrual periods, sterility, signs of estrogen deficiency.

Here again, we see how the activity of a hormone may be evaluated through the changes it causes in the body.

Thus, if you have cellulitis on the inner thighs or arms, especially on the right, and are inclined to develop variably dense lumps in the breasts, again mainly on the right, and if you are also prone to eczema, psoriasis, or bouts of colitis in the ascending (right) colon, it is very probable that your FSH is on the strong side.

Estrogens also belong in this gonadotropic axis. These are the female hormones that play a role not only in women but also in men, because they are involved in building the body's structure and in modeling behavior.

	Strong estrogenic activity	*Weak estrogenic activity*
Your behavioral tendencies	Rather strong libido.	Decline in libido.
Signs	Soft skin, very lax ligaments, rather large breasts, wide and pale areolas in the breast, thick hair, very long eyelashes, rather high-pitched voice, light violet-colored tonsils; diameter of shoulders is smaller than that of the hips.	Dry wrinkled skin, scaly skin, dry and brittle, hair loss and falling eyelashes, under-developed sense of smell.
Problems	Very heavy periods, greasy skin and oily scalp, puts on weight easily with much subcutaneous fat, strong-smelling sweat, water retention, very lax ligaments, horizontal stretch marks.	Clots present on the first day of menstrual period, or lack of periods.

Here we see that a set of signs can point to an excess rather than a deficiency in estrogen activity.

So, if you have very heavy periods, or even flooding, with soft skin and hair that gets greasy quickly, and if your breasts are quite large, and if you are prone to the kind of surface edema known as cellulite, then the activity of your estrogen is certainly too strong.

Progesterone is a hormone that is important for the female reproductive system because it is an intermediary between estrogens and androgens. Apart from its activities in the menstrual cycle, it is also involved in structuring the body.

	Strong progesterone	*Weak progesterone*
Your behavioral tendencies	Participates in the sexual drive.	Lack of sexual drive.
Signs	Tension and diffuse congestion of the breasts, especially of the upper outer quadrants.	The presence of hard and more or less painful areas in the breasts, localized primarily in their upper outer quadrants, and more marked on the left than on the right breast.
Problems	Premenstrual syndrome from after ovulation up to several days before menstruation; clots towards the end of the periods.	Herpes after ovulation, acne on the face, hair on the face and breasts in women; venous problems in lower limbs; blood clots on the second and third day of the periods.

NB: the presence of clots during menstrual periods always indicates an imbalance between estrogen and progesterone.

Women who lack progesterone activity will be inclined to suffer breast tenderness, more so on the left than the right, and their libido is likely to be low. Experiencing clots on the second and third day of menstruation is a particular feature of progesterone deficiency.

The male hormones (androgens) are important elements of the reproductive system and therefore of the gonadotropic axis. They are produced in both sexes by the genital glands (testes, ovaries) and play an important role in the onset of puberty, menopause, or andropause.

Androgens in consort with estrogens participate in building the body's structure and in modeling behavior.

	Strong androgens	Weak androgens
Your behavioral tendencies	Significant capacity for struggle and endurance; stamina and a virile temperament.	Passivity, lack of direction and effectiveness in life, low self-esteem, lack of motivation, decline in physical strength and ability.
Signs	Scar tissue thick and dense; last phalanx of the fingers short and blunt; the rapid growth of childhood abruptly interrupted; hair dense in armpits and in pubic triangle (pointing upwards), hair thinning at temples; voice deepens; diameter of shoulders is bigger than that of the hips.	Muscle hypotrophy often accompanied by increase in abdominal fat; loss of body hair; sparse growth of beard; very lax ligaments; occasional hot flashes and sweats; fatigability.
Problems	Hirsutism and facial acne in women; menstrual disorders.	Erectile dysfunction in men, weak night and morning erection, reduced volume of ejaculate; lowered stamina.

We can see the effects when male hormones are predominant compared with female hormones: the individual has large shoulders and a narrow pelvis, short fingers, coarse pubic hairs (with the pubic triangle pointing toward the umbilicus), receding hairline (hair thinning at the temples), in both men and women, but more commonly in men, menstrual disorders in women and a tendency to facial acne in both men and women.

It is important to make a distinction between the male hormones produced by the genital glands (testes and ovaries) and those produced by the adrenal gland (DHEA). The behavior of individuals in which the activity of male hormones of adrenal origin is predominant is characterized by a desire for power, and is expressed by a combative style with a tendency to confrontation. At its extreme, this imbalance leads to dictatorial and tyrannical behavior.

We now turn to the study of the third axis, the *thyroid axis*. This is the axis that manages the production of all the energy required to build up the body and fight against aggression and respond to stress. We start at the highest level of central control with thyrotropin-releasing hormone (TRH).

	Strong TRH	*Weak TRH*
Your behavioral tendencies	Impulsivity, sudden bursts of energy but with a tendency to anxiety and nervousness.	Poor self-esteem, sexual disorders, difficulty relating to others.
Signs	Brisk reflexes and very narrowed pupils; startled at the slightest noise or approach; tremor of hands, rapid blinking of eyelids; very vivid dreams in color.	Muscle wasting with significant weight loss (see indirect signs of thyroid deficiency).
Problems	Heightened imagination with a tendency to lose contact with reality, risk of delirium.	See indirect signs of thyroid deficiency; in extremis, anorexia nervosa alternating with crises of bulimia.

The clinical manifestations induced by this hormone serve effectively as a measure of the capacity to mobilize energy quickly. When strong, it releases almost undiluted energy, as evidenced by the liveliness of reflexes and the tremors, corroborated by the hyperactive mental states, which spill over into a night of restless dreams in color. If you experience all these signs, your TRH hormone is probably very active.

Besides TRH, the *thyroid gland* is under the control of another hormone, and that is thyroid stimulating hormone (TSH).

The thyroid is the body's heater, since it manages all the oxidations that occur within it. You can recognize its role by the effects it induces in the body.

	Strong thyroid	Weak thyroid
Your behavioral tendencies	Great vivacity.	A general sluggishness, both psychic and physical with reduced genital drive.
Signs	Rapid heart rate, slight tremor of extremities, thick hair, thin eyebrows, long eyelashes, redness in face and palms of hands; sweats easily and doesn't tolerate heat well.	Intolerance and great sensitivity to the cold; skin dry and cold; thin hair, fragile and falling out; eyebrows sparse at their ends; thin brittle nails break easily; voice: low, weak, and hoarse.
Problems	Increase in the size of the thyroid gland; thyroid nodules; excessive sweating; lighter, shorter menstrual periods; generalized itching; diarrhea; irritability; weight loss despite a good appetite; premenstrual syndrome with increased irritability.	Presence of a goiter, accumulation of fluid in the legs; tendency to constipation; hoarseness; weight gain, lack of energy, depressive tendency; heavy periods.

From this table you can see whether you have problems with your thyroid gland. If its activity is too low, you are likely to be overcautious with dry skin and brittle nails, and a low hoarse voice. You will have very heavy periods, and a marked tendency to constipation. Your neck is likely to be swollen.

Let us now consider the hormones belonging to the *somatotropic axis*, the axis in charge of nutrition and construction. Just as we have to put gasoline into an engine for it to work, so for the body to function at all we have to get glucose inside the cells, as well as proteins, fats and other nutrients from our diet. This role is undertaken by the somatotropic axis with hormones specialized for doing just this job; among them *prolactin* plays a major role.

	Strong prolactin	*Weak prolactin*
Your behavioral tendencies	Associated with strong maternal feelings and lowered libido and also a certain kind of emotional detachment, even coldness;[4] lacking imagination and creativity; fearfulness and poor adaptation to stress. May be associated with obsessions and compulsions.	Absence of maternal feelings, fatigue, depression, lack of sexual drive.
Signs	Soft, pale and milky skin; breasts often large and dense with large areolas and large and prominent nipples; heels cracked and swollen, feet often with fallen arches. Involved with the regulation of the transport of water and minerals across cells membranes and into tissues; plays an important role in immunity. Involved as its name suggests in the production of breast milk and in maintaining lactation.	Breasts under-developed, irregular menstrual cycles.
Problems	During the latter part (luteal phase) of the menstrual cycle, women may feel a strong urge to tidy up and organize. Strong prolactin may cause milk to rise before ovulation or before menstruation and may stop periods altogether. Phantom pregnancy. Osteoporosis as well as amenorrhea. Inhibits sexual drive in men. Purulent acne with copious pus; boils. Tends to promote autoimmune pathologies such as rheumatoid arthritis and can act as a growth factor in some cancers by promoting the growth of new blood vessels (angiogenesis).	Suppresses lactation; weight gain; in extremis, severe depressive disorders.

If you are a very maternal, stay-at-home sort of person, and suffer from water retention, especially around your ankles, and with flat feet, and perhaps have very light or absent periods, the odds are that you have strong prolactin. Even more so if any infection produces a lot of pus. If you have been found to have osteoporosis then these signs, taken altogether, indicate high rather than low prolactin.

Insulin plays a crucial role in nutrition because it is the only hormone with the ability to transport glucose from the bloodstream into the cells and so is the major supplier of energy. Also, by regulating the availability of other nutrients, insulin plays an important role in the maintenance of the body's structure. It allows for the storage of energy and favors the laying down of fatty tissue, especially in the abdomen. A fatty pad just above the navel is a sure sign of insulin activity.

As it is the only hormone able to lower blood sugar, it opposes the action of hormones that have the opposite effect. You will now appreciate how, in a world where the individual is bombarded with constant demands, insulin may, in the long run, become exhausted by trying to keep up the supply of energy into the cells, leaving the door wide open to diabetes.

	Strong insulin	*Weak insulin*
Your behavioral tendencies	Shapes your eating behavior.	Shapes your eating behavior.
Signs	Soft but pliable abdomen with fat above the navel. Profuse sweats, with a craving for sugar, yet constantly hungry; high body mass index, reduced potassium and magnesium in blood tests. Diminished Leptin secretion by fat cells makes satiety elusive and so makes it difficult to know when to stop eating.	Decreased appetite.

(Continued)

	Strong insulin	*Weak insulin*
Problems	Weight gain, obesity, high blood sugar most of the time, pre-diabetes, diabetes.	Chronic fatigue, brain fog, fibromyalgia, low blood sugar spells (hypoglycemia), acetone production, leptin resistance.

The unique character of each terrain

The different hormonal systems we've been looking operate together permanently and so constantly react with one another. We must therefore evaluate all physical signs according to their interrelationships, as well as in their own right, if we want to have a clear understanding of the exact state of the terrain.

The patient's state is always a mosaic of signs that is specific to each individual. The expertise of the doctor in charge of a case should try and follow the logic of the mechanisms that led to the disruption of a particular terrain, looking for the common thread, trying to shed light on how diseases may evolve, and so be able to personalize the treatment of each patient.

To illustrate the intricate relationships between the many different hormones and their relations with the autonomic nervous system, let us take as an example a woman with a complex set of signs that demonstrate an imbalance due to several associated factors. She is extremely nervous, anxious, and emotionally very sensitive who is prone to palpitations. She complains of many other symptoms: constipation, excessive timidity, premenstrual tension, cellulite, cold hands, lumps in the breasts, and much else besides. Everything gets worse at the full moon and when the season changes, and, of course, before her periods. All these signs can be attributed to a hyper-functioning of the alpha-sympathetic system, the thyroid, and estrogens. Unless her functional disturbances are properly resolved, she runs a real risk of developing serious gynecological problems in the future, such as tumors in her breast, fibroids, ovarian cysts, and even develop a condition like rheumatoid arthritis.

There is a complex logic at work in the body of every individual. The hormones which shape and act on it should do so in a way that is in overall coordination. Some terrains are more prone to certain diseases. They should be monitored very carefully in the interests of a truly preventative medicine. First of all, the terrain needs to be clearly identified so that corrective measures can be established. Take, for example, a person whose response to all kinds of stress, including emotional and psychological stress, is excessive. The hyperactivity of their growth factors coupled with a high-octane surge from their thyroid subjects their body to a constant state of overdrive. If this coincides with low immunity, they will be much more likely to develop a rapidly progressive disorder than someone with low immunity but without these other characteristics. There is huge potential for this approach for anyone concerned about his or her health, who is prepared to adopt a personalized program adapted to the unique characteristics of their terrain. These are important aims and objectives of Endobiogenic medicine.

CHAPTER SIX

Medicinal plants: real promise or false dawn?

Notes from a patient

It is easy to get the impression from articles in the popular press or from books hyped by the media that everybody has rediscovered the healing power of plants. All of a sudden, they can cure everything! While they have largely been abandoned by pharmaceutical companies as a source of promising new drugs, and effectively banned from therapeutic use by French law,[1] they are making a comeback in the popular imagination. It must be said that this enthusiasm for back-to-nature is a recurrent theme. We perennially turn towards some idealized source to heal all our ills. Now it is the turn of plants to offer a solution for everything. Herb teas, decoctions of roots, and capsules of herbal powder are said to complement or even offer a realistic alternative to synthetic medicines.

In 2012 the public showed as great a hunger for natural alternatives as they did in the 1970s.[2] On June 10, 2010, the cover of *Le Point*, a mass-market French magazine, featured "A Guide to Healing Plants." On page one, we have a nutritionist basking in some rural idyll, with her basket full of plants, seasonal fruits and vegetables. All smiles, she recommends 12 plants that no home should be without. The huge interest shown by patients (and some doctors) in these "plants that are good for us" can partly be put down to anxiety about the side effects of certain drugs, heightened by scandals associated with their promotion and use. The headline in an article about Mediator® that appeared in *Le Nouvel Observateur* read "Death By Prescription." A climate of suspicion on the potential dangers of synthetic medicinal products began to emerge. At the same time, those who were opposed to modern medicine rode on a wave of confidence as if the hour of "disenchantment" was at hand, and might signal the demise of miracle drugs. At the same time, the appeal of natural pharmacy, which apparently had worked "small miracles" in so many patients, seemed irresistible. How heartwarming to return to nature! All one has to do is to get to know the plants better and to find the ones that would sort out our symptoms. These ready-made prescriptions are so easy to pick up in supermarkets or pharmacies. So simple and natural, they can soothe all our daily ills, and with no real side effects.

In the past, whenever I had a headache, I would reach for the paracetamol! For heartburn and stomach problems I would immediately take a Motilium® or an antacid. Now, I feel much better off with plants. And for a given symptom, instead of waiting for an appointment to see a doctor, from the first signs, it is enough to do a Google search and click on "healing plants," or call my girlfriend, who knows everything about natural products, and I discover the miracle solution.

Like many others, I make the most of all the little health secrets revealed in magazines or on television. I comb through all the formulas in books written by various naturopaths in which they freely share their tips and anecdotes. As a result, I feel better informed and so can ask my pharmacist if the need arises for such and such a plant to treat an infection or another one to restore my energy or help me sleep better, or whatever. During the drearier seasons, I no longer think twice about buying supplements to perk me up so that I can live life more fully. Then there are all these plants supposed to hydrate your skin before you take a holiday in the sun, and on it goes. Pharmacy shelves heave with miracle plant-based products that promise "inner beauty," or which will enrich your complexion and do wonders for the circulation to your legs. There they are, calling to me, from the counter, close to the till. My friends and I are tempted to try them out.

We pass on the address of the latest fashionable naturopath; we talk about the latest plant that enabled a friend to get through the entire winter in remarkably good shape. We share our grandmothers' secrets; they knew how to make the best use of infusions of particular plants. We convince ourselves and so give into the allure of these so-called "natural" products flooding the pharmacies. Anyway, they can't do you any harm, can they? Yet, in spite of our enthusiasm, we return to the same questions: are these plants as effective as synthetic medicaments? What can they really treat or prevent? Are we not falling for the myth of the magical elixir? To what extent has their use come under scientific research and scrutiny? I put all these questions to Dr. Lapraz. Here is what he had to say by way of reply.

Beware of rogue herbal medicine

Just because medical drugs and chemotherapy are potent and are open to misuse, it doesn't at all follow that medicinal plants are innocuous and their use in Phytotherapy is entirely without risk. Ignorance about how plants act on the body has been implicated in a number of cases of harmful outcomes caused by the inappropriate use of herbal medicine. Immediate adverse reactions are not unknown but, more often than not, the harm is more insidious because adverse effects may be latent; showing up later makes them hard to attribute. The full extent of this problem has not yet been researched. The untutored use of plants can lead to a range of problems: wrong dosage, interactions with drugs, and the inappropriate choice of plants for want of a reliable diagnosis. Seduced by alternative medicine ads, people take plant-based products that are quite inappropriate for their condition or take high doses in pursuit of a desired outcome, and so run the risk of overdosing. Unsuspecting patients may take medicinal plants at the same as their prescription drugs, without realizing that such a combination could potentially cause greatly endanger their health.

Natural Health practitioners are often ignorant of the complex actions of the plants they prescribe and their real effects on their patient's condition. Unless a precise diagnosis is made, these plants can cause a lot of harm, without anyone being aware of it. Such problems may occur a long time after the course of treatment, and will never be traced back to the plant-based prescription. These practitioners have not necessarily been trained in pharmacology and the chemistry of plants and so will not be able to advise their patients competently as to whether their Phytotherapeutic treatment can be taken concurrently with prescription drugs. Thus, their patients may run a serious risk of plant–drug interaction.

That medicinal plants are potentially toxic is beyond question, despite the claims and denials of suppliers, who want to sell their products, come what may. Of course, by saying this, I am not implying that there are any deliberate attempts to harm anyone. Hunters have exploited toxic sap to kill their prey (such as curare on arrow heads) and history records some notorious poisoners who knew exactly how deadly certain plants were. I am not referring to plants that have long been well known for their powerful and fatal side effects; this, of course, is not our concern with the medicinal plants that are in current use.

Nonetheless, all plants, including those sold over the counter or listed in the pharmacopeia, may be harmful in a much more subtle way, and by very different mechanisms. These we will touch on later. We must also make a distinction between side effects from the wrong prescription, or an unsuitable dosage or non-compliance by the patient on the one hand, and those related to a particular sensitivity or to a pathology not yet picked up in the patient, on the other.

The temptation of a higher dose

The toxicity of a plant is mostly down to taking higher than the recommended dose, and consumers can get carried away by exaggerated advertising claims. It is easy be swayed by the inflated promises and assurances made in this kind of material: "this plant creates mental harmony without being addictive"; another is claimed to be more effective than its conventional medical equivalent and yet another has proven benefits in weight loss. And how tempting to sample plants from exotic lands that are "endowed by nature with wonderful properties," from Asia, Tibet, or from the deserts of Mexico. All the more so when it is claimed that they will make you lose weight in a few days, without any effort; or they will "dramatically restore lost vitality and restore sexual vigor"!

But when the desired effect fails to materialize, patients may succumb to the temptation to increase the dose by drinking more of the herbal tea or increasing the number of capsules. Convinced that the plant is harmless, they exceed the prescribed dose, and the adverse effects soon follow: upset gut with allergies, as well as hormonal and nervous disorders. A common risk with these dubious preparations is that they are a combination of too many plants. Inevitably these will entail conflicting properties and are likely to have the opposite effect than the one intended.

The reality of plant–drug interactions

It is important to be aware of the very real harm that may be caused by interactions between prescription drugs and medicinal plants. It is very common and is a cause of great concern for those of us who work in this field. We do not have any accurate data about the size and extent of the problem. The active principles of medicinal plants may significantly modify the behavior of synthetic drugs. Here are a few examples:

A patient taking simvastatin to reduce cholesterol may not know that the grapefruit juice he drinks daily will increase the absorption of this medicinal product by a factor of 15[3] resulting in an overdose and an increased risk of developing side effects, especially in the muscles. On the other hand, if he had taken St. John's wort, commonly used as a "natural" antidepressant, this would have had the opposite effect, making the simvastatin less effective!

Both St. John's wort and grapefruit juice increase the rate of the breakdown in the liver of Indinavir (Crixivan), a drug used in the treatment of AIDS; being eliminated faster makes the drug less effective. But juice has the opposite effects on other drugs used in the treatment of AIDS. By slowing the breakdown of Saquinavir (Invirase), the drug accumulates to unacceptable levels. All these effects make the care of the sick more complicated. Grapefruit can also interact with many other drugs such as some anti-hypertensive and anti-allergic agents, and tranquilizers.

The example of these two plants shows the caution needed when mixing plants with conventional medicines. A patient who is already on a cocktail of drugs may be persuaded to take some herbs, with the thought that if they don't do any good, at least they can't do any harm. you can be sure that if there are any effects, the patient's doctor will have great difficulty in making sense of them. There must be so many other phenomena of this kind that we just don't know about.

Many food plants affect the rate at which the blood clots, either by increasing or decreasing it, as do herbs sold over the counter or as so-called dietary supplements. This fact has great significance for patients taking anticoagulant drugs. These are prescribed for cardiovascular conditions to reduce the risk of stroke. Garlic, for example, tends to elevate the INR (international normalized ratio),[4] and so can increase the risk of hemorrhage. Other plants can alter the rate at which the body metabolizes a drug, either speeding it up or slowing it down. They do so in a number of ways: by interfering with liver function, or by making fundamental changes in the metabolism or in the management of the body by the endocrine system.

Do not play sorcerer's apprentice with essential oils

While essential oils are very popular, perhaps few people who use them realize the risks they may run by ill-advised self-medication. These are very active products, which are active even at low doses, and their effects can show up quickly in anyone, depending on their health. To give an example, you wouldn't recommend essential oils of rosemary, oregano, or marjoram to an asthmatic given that these plants stimulate the parasympathetic system, which would cause a reduction in the diameter of the bronchi. This would obstruct the flow of oxygen into the lungs, and so precipitate an asthmatic crisis. But who will be there to make the connection? Similarly, are there adequate cautions for women who may be advised to take the essential oils of caraway, cypress, garden angelica, or sage? The strong estrogenic activity of these plants puts women with a tendency to hyper-estrogenism at great risk of exacerbating this hormonal imbalance, and so are contraindicated in such cases? Who is going to warn a man suffering from an enlarged prostate about the risk of urine retention from taking the essential oils of wild thyme, cypress, and thyme that he was advised to take for his bronchitis? The action of these oils on the autonomic nervous system may cause a blockage of the urethral sphincter. Who knows that the essential oils of nutmeg and hyssop can trigger epileptic seizures in susceptible people?

This huge problem of interactions should be addressed with the utmost caution, but is unfortunately dismissed by some practitioners, as is attested by one of my patients who was being treated at the hospital for her polyarthritis. When she asked her specialist if she could continue taking her plant-based treatment at the same time as the anti-inflammatory drugs he was prescribing, he replied, without even asking me what she was taking: "No problem, Ma'am, do just as you like; it doesn't matter, because, in any event, it can't do you any harm!" A most disturbing answer. Shouldn't the doctor have enquired about the exact nature of the plant-based products she was taking, and in light of their interaction might he not reconsider his own prescription?

However, this attitude is by no means uncommon even in specialties such as oncology where the stakes are so high. Oncologists are so accustomed to using their powerful treatments that they cannot imagine that plants could have any comparable effect on their patients. They are quite unaware that plants could influence how the drugs activity on the body and thus alter the progress of the disease. And so, they reassure their patients with the usual formula: "well, do whatever you want, even if it does not help, it cannot hurt you anyway."

The dangers of amateurism: a tragic case

Certain "natural health practitioners," who have received no formal medical education, prescribe plants empirically where the desired outcome is based on traditional use. There are schools that enroll people on crash courses consisting of a number of "weekend seminars," in which they claim to train students to a level of competence in all the techniques and methods, whereas 7 years in medical school are hardly enough to equip the trainee doctor to go into medical practice. This raises thorny ethical problems: where does responsibility lie for those who, without formal qualification, make a living from giving advice on health matters? Patient management and the prescription of medicinal plants require a good level of medical education. Without it, all manner of abuses become possible when these practitioners, in all good faith, believe they cannot be wrong because they use only natural products.

One of our colleagues from Saint Antony's Hospital told us a tragic tale about a patient who had experienced vaginal bleeding some years after her menopause. She had read in a magazine that Salad Burnet is good for bleeding, so she decided to give it a try as she assumed her symptom was benign. Her naturopath, who had no formal medical training, reassured her and promised that if she took a herbal tea she would be cured in eight days, which is just what happened, as predicted. Two months later, she started bleeding again, but now much more heavily. The patient went for a second time to see her naturopath who told her to drink 3 liters of a very concentrated infusion each day of three herbs with a reputation for stopping periods. But this time progress was much slower: she continued to hemorrhage, though much less heavily, which reassured her. Then, she started to experience lower back pain, especially at night. As she had suffered from lumbago for many years, she didn't pay too much attention and just put up with it. Nevertheless, she went back to her naturopath because the pain was becoming more severe and persistent. The naturopath recommended her to a famous bonesetter, who was said to be "so good that people come from the far corners of the country to see him, with busloads and ambulances parked outside his practice." This celebrated healer greeted her then, with his pendulum in his right hand, he placed his left hand on the patient's painful vertebrae. He said he had found the ones that were jammed and needed adjusting and with a sudden snap and crack, he announced: "There you go, I have released them!" The diagnosis was made by a laying on of hands to "search for energy imbalances." With one glance, this was confirmed: the glands are functioning poorly, mainly the thyroid and in the colon. The prescription was written on a letterhead listing numerous titles: iridologist, specialist in hygiene and natural medicine, radiesthesia, spinal manipulation, and colon cleansing.

The patient was reassured. She took the new plants prescribed conscientiously, which were supposed to get her back on her feet. Unfortunately, six weeks later, a catastrophic hemorrhage almost carried her off. She was taken to the emergency ward of the hospital where the intern on duty made the diagnosis in less than ten seconds. All it needed was for him to insert a speculum to discover cancer of the uterus in a very advanced stage, the tumor having already reached the spine. Sad to relate that the choices made by this woman led to her very painful death, and unnecessary because this kind of tumor would have been easily picked up by a gynecologist. A delay in diagnosis is always prejudicial because it deprives the patient of an effective and personalized treatment.

It was unfortunate that the plant prescribed by the naturopath was effective in stopping the bleeding. While the effect was real and apparently beneficial, in fact it only served to draw attention away from an early stage uterine cancer and so delayed the diagnosis with tragic consequences. This is the great danger of the non-medical use of medicinal plants: the prescription was based on a symptom, hemorrhage, and not on a diagnosis, a bleeding tumor. Once again, we see the limitations of a purely symptomatic approach, where the plant is matched with a symptom, just as in modern pharmacology, a specific etiology calls for a specific molecule.

In addition, because their "diagnoses" are not based upon anatomical and physiological understanding, non-physicians lack the means to critically review their own practice. It is clear in this tragic case, that the patient was at no time given a clinical examination, which is essential to identify any pathology, and to differentiate between benign or malignant. The referral of this woman to a bonesetter rather than a physician shows how prevalent these unregulated healthcare networks are. The bonesetter's sham consultation makes a mockery of medicine by using words which seem authentic: "glands, thyroid, colon" but which only conceal ignorance. He would be unable to give a scientific explanation for his "findings." Unfortunately, this is not an isolated case. Patients who are convinced that they are doing the right thing by using such practices, more often than not, find that things turn out badly.

In effect, such a case could reasonably be described as a new form of "natural iatrogenic pathology," as opposed to "chemical iatrogenic pathology," and one that is directly related to the use, or rather misuse, of plants, and to the lack of training in the one who prescribed them.

Beware of charlatans

There is a regressive trend towards magical primitivism exemplified by a belief in "the mysterious therapeutic power of plants," a power that escapes rational explanation. There have always been stories of extraordinary cures, in which hopeless cases are miraculously cured by imbibing special herbal brews. Such tales open the door to superstition and has nothing to do with science. Having treated thousands of patients for 40 years with medicinal plants on a daily basis, I can assure you that I have yet to meet with a miracle, as defined in the dictionary: "an event not explicable by natural laws and which is attributed to a divine power.[5]"

On the contrary, in my Clinical Phytotherapy practice I witnessed amazing results in serious cases, time and time again. These spurred me on to clinical research, to try to understand the physiological mechanisms responsible for such outcomes. Some patients unfortunately are more likely to seek out a natural healer with no medical training or an unconventional doctor who, casting the net wide, will prescribe esoteric nostrums, based on energy or quantum medicine, or some other type of gobbledygook. Such of these astonishing potpourris are formulated in a way that which may attract the uncritical or naive patient. But if the public is gullible enough to go for this sort of thing, is it not because medicine rejects out of hand any practice or approach that is not based on the prescription chemical medicinal products?

The abandonment of plants by medicine and the denial of their efficacy has been a major contribution to their marginalization. This view has become so commonplace that patients are surprised to find that a physician trained in Phytotherapy relies on laboratory tests to support the diagnosis. Indeed, the idea of herbal medicine as outside scientific disciplines is so ingrained that the patient may not realize that the tools available to modern medical science are indispensable for prescribing a course of treatment that is based on plants. For us, however, Clinical Phytotherapy has always been a branch of medicine. It fulfills all its requirements, beginning with the examination of the patient, coming to a diagnosis, monitoring the outcomes of the treatment, and following-up the development of every case. Any general practitioner should be able to offer his or her patients a plant-based treatment as an alternative. To achieve this, it is absolutely necessary to reintegrate the study of medicinal plants into the curriculum in medical schools.

When practiced properly, Phytotherapy is not a fashion, but a necessity. A good example of herbal medicine as public health policy is provided by Mexico City where the political, administrative, and medical bodies adopted Clinical Phytotherapy in their healthcare system, in clinics and healthcare centers.[6]

Beware of self-medication using plant-based products

- In the absence of a medical diagnosis, you run the risk of missing underlying disease.
- Without accurate medical diagnosis, the prescription of a medicinal plant can be hazardous.
- Without fully understanding the patient's condition, the prescription of a medicinal plant can produce the opposite effects to those intended.
- Without a deep understanding of the properties of plants, harm may be caused by using them indiscriminately.
- We should use critical judgment about the use of any plant that is claimed to be a panacea.
- All formulations should be accompanied by instructions for use and precautions about usage.
- Pressure from advertisers should be resisted when it comes to the indiscriminate consumption of plant-based dietary supplements, herbal products, and antioxidants, whether over the counter or on the internet.

Clinical phytotherapy: new opportunities

Why were medicinal plants abandoned in favor of synthetic drugs?

An idea prevalent today deems it sufficient to remove the symptoms of disease to consider the patient healed. Towards this end, pharmaceutical research has developed molecules that are precisely formulated to have a very specific and targeted action on the body. As we'll see, this is the main reason that has led to abandonment of plants in medical practice.

Medicinal plants have always been with us: their use is as old as humankind. In all civilizations and at all times, people have used them to care for the sick and there is abundant prehistoric evidence for their ubiquitous use. Early historical records, such as cuneiform tablets and papyrus scrolls, testify to their early use in Mesopotamia and in Egypt. The Vedic tradition in India was mostly oral but medical and surgical texts survive from the time of Gautama Buddha (560–480 BCE).[7] In China, the most ancient texts have been lost, but are dated to about 500 BCE. An unbroken written record survives intact from 500 CE and attests to a tradition that was already a 1000 years old. In the Mediterranean world, Hippocrates—the so-called "father of medicine"—discusses the effects of plants on the sick. During the same classical era in Athens, Theophrastus (372–287 BCE), a colleague and younger contemporary of Aristotle, wrote the foundation texts in botanical science and is deservedly accorded the accolade of the "Father of Botany."[8] Although he was not an herbalist, he provided the framework in which plants could be discussed scientifically. He associated with a celebrated physician called Diocles who is credited with writing the first Greek herbal, though only fragments survive. The first professional physician to describe himself as a herbalist was Cretaus (c.120–60 BCE) but it is Dioscorides (c.40–90 CE) who is best known. His *De materia medica*, in which he describes the medicinal use of over 500 plants, remained in use as a reference book until the eighteenth century. Even this is eclipsed by the encyclopedic works of surgery, medicine, and pharmacy by the prodigious Galen of Pergamum (c.130–c.201CE) who was personal physician to the Roman Emperor Marcus Aurelius. He is widely considered to be the "single most influential figure in the history of Western medicine from Roman times to the twentieth century."[9] The development of trade routes to India and Asia and the spread of the great Islamic cultures greatly enriched the knowledge of therapeutic plants. The famous school of Salerno near Naples (*Schola Medica Salernitana*) dominated the Middle Ages where the theoretical and practical education was based on the study of the classical Greek and Latin texts as well as on physical examination of patients. By the year 985, Salerno was awarding the title doctor to its graduates.[10] From 1492, the rich flora and sophisticated pharmacopeia of Mesoamerica contributed enormously to the materia medica of Europe. The many important additions included ipecacuanha, Peruvian bark (which yielded quinine), and balsam of Peru. This influx of plants also had a considerable impact on the diet and culture of Europe with maize, sweet potatoes, potatoes, tomatoes, runner beans, French beans, pineapples, sunflowers, and Jerusalem artichokes coming into cultivation early in the sixteenth century, especially in Italy. Chili peppers, tobacco, and chocolate were evaluated for medicinal benefits. The rise of the scientific method in the seventeenth and the eighteenth centuries led to the growing dominance of experimentation and analytic methods, in keeping with the dominant Age of Reason. The publication in 1735 of *Systema Naturae* by Carl Linnaeus standardized the convention of scientific binomial nomenclature and was the stimulus to the foundation of modern plant and animal biology.

The rise of chemical analytical methods gathered pace during the nineteenth century, so that one discovery followed on the heels of another. Technical progress allowed the complex chemical structure of compounds found in plants to be elucidated. One of the first active principles to be isolated (from the opium poppy) was the alkaloid morphine. This molecule was central to the development of modern analgesics and was first identified in 1804. The plant itself had of course been known since prehistoric times and is mentioned by Homer in the *Iliad*, as an ingredient of *Nepenthe*, the beverage that made one forget sorrow and pain. Intense pharmacological research ensued in a race to identify the many other active compounds in plants. Traditional plant-based therapy was reevaluated as alkaloids and glycosides were identified. These active principles came to be considered more effective, easier to dose, and with more consistent actions than the simple extracts or decoctions used up to that time. Quinine, once a leading anti-malarial medicine, is extracted from the bark of species in the genus *Cinchona*. Colchicine, still a major medication for gout, is derived from the bulb of the autumn crocus (*Colchicum autumnale*); ergotamine, for treating migraine headaches, comes from a fungus known as ergot (*Claviceps purpurea*) that infects rye; curare, with potent muscle relaxant properties, comes from species of Amazonian lianas in the genus *Strychnos*. Digoxin, one of the most important substances in the treatment of cardiac failure, is obtained from the leaves of common foxglove (*Digitalis purpurea*). Aspirin, perhaps the most utilized medicine in the world, is synthesized from salicylic acid, derived from salicin, which is found in the bark of the willow tree (*Salix alba*) and in the flowering tops of meadowsweet (*Filipendula ulmaria*). The alkaloids obtained from the leaves of the Madagascar periwinkle (*Catharanthus roseus*) enter into the composition of several highly potent chemotherapy agents used today in the treatment of cancer.

Chemistry, then, was the royal road to medicine and removed a certain aura of mystery that had enshrouded plants. In spite of the fact that up to the Second World War most medicinal products came from plants, it was chemistry and not any appeal to magical powers that determined their effectiveness. Henceforward, this would be resolved by the analysis of material compounds and represents a break with thousands of years of empirical knowledge. Countless studies have been conducted, both on animals and on isolated tissues or organs, to try to understand how plant metabolites exert their effects on living organisms.

Isolating the active principle of the plants: the triumph of the single molecule

Studies have shown that the character and concentration of the natural chemical compounds found in plants vary considerably depending on the season, and the place and time of harvest. Plants are indeed alive, and in common with all living organisms, their metabolism is in a constant state of flux, and so their metabolic products vary over time. For example, the essential oil produced by common or garden thyme (*Thymus vulgaris*) contains thymol in concentrations that can vary from 25% to 40%, depending on whether it is harvested in the morning or in the evening. There may be hundreds of compounds found in a single plant, so this variability in their composition poses a great challenge to researchers, especially as some of the effects these active principles cause are also variable. In an attempt to simplify and clarify this highly complex situation, there was an understandable trend towards studying the effects of only those compounds found in large quantities in the plant. Once isolated, the compound was assumed to be responsible for the action observed in the experimental subject. They then calculated the dose that would be needed to obtain the desired effect and standardized that dose so that it would be deemed appropriate for any individual.

But, as plants do not produce consistent levels of these major active principles, they cannot be relied upon to achieve a reproducible action, in the way that modern pharmacology requires. As a result, researchers stopped using plants at all and took the simpler and easier route of reproducing the well-defined single molecule. Thus, they gradually developed simple products, with a defined chemical structure, first by hemi-synthesis, and then shortly afterwards, by the total synthesis of compounds not actually found in the original plant. In this way, an industry grew up committed to developing standardized products and prescribing them indiscriminately for all sick individuals, without taking into account the unique and particular characteristics of each person. The ability of plant medicines with their broad and extensive reach within the human body was replaced by the precise and potent action of chemical medicinal compounds. These were much easier to manipulate and control in contrast to the complex material from plants, which was variable in composition and more difficult to manage. Plant medicines were brushed aside and fell into disuse. Not only were the plants lost but with them went the integrative approach that attempts always to match the disease with the patient in the wholeness of their being.

Soon, the race towards greater efficiency accelerated. The hunt was on for spectacular and lucrative success with the development of new and more potent products with targeted action. The goal to develop and refine the molecule that would block the expression of disease was reinforced by the therapeutic successes that resulted from this approach. Given this prevailing orthodoxy, the place of the plant in the therapeutic arsenal no longer made sense, and could not be justified. These new and extremely potent medicinal products relegated plants to the status of quaint remnants from an outmoded past. The study of the therapeutic properties of plants was therefore no longer seen as relevant by medical science, and so, removed from the curriculum, was no longer taught to medical students.

However, it was not long before the pitfalls of modern medicine became apparent: wide generalizations and narrow focus produce their own problems. The blanket prescription of potent molecules to whole populations that should have been reserved for the small percentage of patients who really needed them is at the heart of the current crisis in medicine. Medical research is directed towards reliable remedies with reproducible (and therefore generalizable) effects. This favors synthetic medicinal compounds, which have the additional advantage of being integrated within the manufacturing and production processes of their paymasters, Big Pharma.

Doctors, placed as they are between the producer and consumer, are more likely to use products that are more convenient to use. Besides, if they are only interested in treating the manifestations of disease, they would be inclined to take the easier option rather than use medicinal plants, from which the real benefit can only be obtained when the doctor addresses the imbalances hidden beneath the disease.

This state of affairs is the inevitable consequence of an extreme reductionist approach that reduces phenomena as complex as the functioning of living organisms to their constituent parts. Such is the direction taken by research scientists: this exclusively analytical approach fragments the unity of the plant into its many diverse constituents. It is time to turn the tide and to reconsider the immense therapeutic opportunities offered by plants to the sick as well as to those in good health. Trivialized as "domestic remedies" by those who have no understanding or experience of their use, they are so often dismissed by policy-makers in the sphere of public health. The challenge facing modern medicine is to reintegrate the entirety of the human being with the management of disease and to reunify the totality of the whole plant with its therapeutic use.

For the reintegration of the medicinal plants in conventional medicine

A return to the medical use of plants should not be a regression to previous practice. They should be used in an entirely different manner than that employed prior to their exclusion medical practice.

As my colleague Christian Duraffourd and I have stated in an article published in the journal *Enjeux du monde*, "Our interest in Phytotherapy is not in any way a response to a 'back-to-nature' fad, or based upon some sort of mythical belief in the 'miraculous powers' of herbs. It is born from the day-to-day practice of medicine and the careful observation of the real needs of patients and the solutions offered by medicinal plants."[11]

We therefore need to rethink the place of plants in medical practice, to reintegrate them into the heart of the therapeutic project in a progressive and balanced way. This will require those who use them to respect the rules governing any medical treatment, from which of course medicinal plants are by no means exempt.

The whole plant rather than its active principle

The prescription of whole-plant extracts has the great advantage over that of isolated active ingredients in that they produce a rounder, more comprehensive effect on the patient. This more desirable action alone justifies their use. By way of illustration, let us take the example of artichoke.

Artichoke is a plant traditionally used to improve digestion. We eat parts of the flower-head as a vegetable, but it is the leaf that is used in medicine. Total leaf extracts lower the level of cholesterol, are diuretic, and are cholagogues, which means that they favor the evacuation of bile, an action amply corroborated by modern research.[12] The leaves contain several acidic compounds: malic, succinic, and citric acids, but in isolation, none of them taken separately has a diuretic or cholagogue effect comparable to that of the whole-plant extracts of artichoke.

This finding reflects the fact that the various constituents in the plant act in synergy, each reinforcing the action of the others. The whole plant acts comprehensively on the body thanks to this combination effect with all the active principles in harmonious balance. Doctors who have practiced Clinical Phytotherapy for 40-odd years have gained a clear insight into this synergistic action of the whole plant when treating their patients. They have a considerable advantage over their predecessors, who practiced Phytotherapy in previous centuries, as they now have at their disposal all the analytical techniques of modern science to validate or invalidate their clinical observations. These radiological and biological techniques will permit the actions of medicinal plants to be measured objectively and put the facts beyond dispute. Numerous examples of such investigations will be given in Chapter 7 "The Growing International Influence of Clinical Phytotherapy."

The need for definition and quality assurance of herbal material

When you look into the medicinal plants on the market that can freely be bought over the counter by anyone, you will be aghast at the danger to which people in search of treatment expose themselves. Given the dubious claims made for products of unreliable quality and unspecified origin, people wanting to use medicinal plants ought to apply several essential tests according to the following criteria.

The first criterion requires the exclusive use of certified therapeutic grade herbal material. This implies the traceability of the plant from the producer to prescriber and patient. It is essential to know exactly where and how the plant was grown and for it to be authenticated as botanically correct. Its production should be subject to quality control, and guaranteed free from contamination by pests or pesticides, nitrates, or heavy metals. Quality assurance of the finished product should monitor the consistency of its content in active principles and the stability of the pharmaceutical formulation, whether a mother tincture, a dry or fluid extract, or a nebulized product. These products should have been assessed for bioavailability and certified as fit for therapeutic use, having complied with all the protocols of quality control. Without such assurance, the effectiveness of the treatment may be compromised, even if the prescription has been properly and correctly formulated. Furthermore, unexpected side effects can appear from low quality plant material.

Given all these variables, the development of safe phyto-medicines is of great importance. As a case in point, the use of microspheres[13] allows for a very uniform release of active ingredients as compared with the powdered plant, for which the rate of distribution of the active substance to the tissues is too random and variable.

In September, 2011, a study was conducted in West Africa, using microspheres, on the efficacy and safety of a local plant *Hymenocardia acida* (Euphorbiaceae) for the treatment of hypertension.[14] The trial, which compared the efficacy of the plant extract with that of Amlodipine (one of a number of drugs used in the treatment of essential hypertension), demonstrated a significant decrease in systolic and diastolic pressure in hypertensive patients over the whole range of severity. Authorized for sale in Africa at a remarkably low cost, this phyto-medicine, marketed as Guinex HTA, made a very effective Phytotherapeutic product available at low cost in developing countries, in place of expensive products, which these countries could not afford.

The second criterion that needs to be observed before embarking on any course of treatment is to understand what effects it will have on the body, and plants are not exempt from this rule. You cannot hope to treat a patient's condition using plant prescriptions without first having a thorough and detailed knowledge of their physiological properties. Thus, if we want to reduce the activity of the alpha-sympathetic system, we must use a plant that has the property of slowing it down. We cannot be satisfied with prescribing plants that are reputed to have some generalized action on the nervous system: we must know its precise mechanism of action. Once these two requirements have been met, the next step is to formulate a course of treatment.

Clinical dignosis based upon a comprehensive patient-centered approach

No treatment should be undertaken before the patient has received a medical examination, and in this respect plant-based treatments are no different. *Once the quality of the plant material has been assured and the doctor knows what effects to expect, he or she can devise a treatment plan.* There is more than one approach available to those contemplating treatments with medicinal plants. Let us review three of the available options.

The **first** approach is simple and consists in treating the patient's symptoms. The patient has a fever, the doctor prescribes a plant with antipyretic action. If he or she presents symptoms of constipation, the doctor prescribes a laxative plant, for migraine, a plant for treating such headaches, for infection, an anti-microbial plant, and so on. This approach is identical to that followed by conventional medicine, with the difference that the latter employs synthetic medicinal products only. Another difference is that as chemical medicines are so much more powerful than plants, they get faster results and doses are easier to standardize. Certainly, with symptomatic treatment we can achieve positive results using medicinal plants, but much more slowly and with less consistency because their action is not really comparable to that of synthetic remedies. Therefore, when using this approach, one is not comparing Like with Like, so there is no point in comparing plants with medicinal drugs.

The **second** approach is more complex and depends upon using plants for their effects on the organs of detoxification. It is based on the idea that the malfunction of organs such as the liver, intestines, and kidneys has contributed to the disease or to the symptom at least, and so hopes to improve the state of the patient by improving the functioning of these organs. This practice is the so-called drainage method, commonly used by healthcare practitioners. While this approach can certainly achieve positive results, it is not without its limitations: how sure can one be of correctly identifying the organ that needs to be drained? Which of its multiple functions should one take into account, and how long should the treatment last? Perhaps more importantly, this approach fails to address the cause of the organ malfunction. It observes a sign and takes it at face value, without offering an explanation for its appearance. It is imperative to go beyond the observed phenomena and reach for a deeper understanding.

This imperative takes us to the **third** approach: Clinical Phytotherapy, one that is based on the Endobiogenic approach towards the patient. For the group of physicians who use this approach, the limitations of the symptomatic use of medicinal products (whether based on plants or not) are overcome not by changing the means, but by changing the method. This method does not consider the removal of all clinical signs to be its primary task, but rather to take the signs and symptoms as an indication of a deep imbalance, and to find out what has led to this state of affairs in the first place and has allowed it to continue.

The choice of the plants must be based therefore on a detailed appraisal of the terrain on which they will have to operate. A rigorous therapeutic strategy needs to be in place, without falling back on ready-made prescriptions or formulas. Each plant has to be selected, either alone or in combination with other plants, according to a comprehensive evaluation of the state of the patient, as shown in Chapter 4 when we talked about Endobiogeny and presented the case of Marie-Laure. This is a progressive approach in which plants can be used in conjunction with synthetic drugs. It represents a personalized therapeutic strategy and is based on a revolutionary conception of health and disease. Whole-plant extracts are better suited to the physiology of the human body, and a more pharmacologically active treatment should be prescribed only if the body is unable to respond to the active principles from plants, for example, when the dosage is too low or in cases where the body lacks the capacity to respond.

While doctors who follow the Endobiogenic approach treat their patients mainly with medicinal plants, they may also have recourse to other natural products, such as micronutrients, clay, seawater, lactobacilli, pollen, and a range of other therapeutic agents. Massage and thermal treatments as well as personalized dietary regimes all have a part to play in a comprehensive approach to the treatment of the terrain.

Three golden rules for the medical use of plants

1. Practitioners should have received formal education and training in medicine and should have a comprehensive knowledge of medicinal plants and their properties.
2. Medicinal plants should be administered only after thorough diagnostic evaluation of the patient's terrain has been made by a broader approach than the purely symptomatic.
3. Medicinal plants should be administered as whole extracts and with well-defined objectives and intended outcomes, while reducing the risk of unwanted effects to a minimum.

CHAPTER SEVEN

The growing international influence of clinical phytotherapy

In 1993, Professor Rachid Chemli, Dr. Christian Duraffourd, and I organized the first "Intercontinental Congress on Medicinal Plants and Phytotherapy." It was convened in Tunisia and brought together 500 participants from 49 different countries: doctors, pharmacists, researchers, members of international organizations and industry, associative movements, and NGOs.

A number of French doctors[1] contributed to the great success of this congress. They presented over one hundred case histories in which Clinical Phytotherapy achieved very good results. The cases covered a wide range of pathologies, including asthma, bronchitis, sinusitis, acne, psoriasis, eczema, shingles, high cholesterol, diabetes, hepatitis, osteoarthritis, cystitis, adenoma of the prostate, sterility, premenstrual syndrome, migraine, insomnia, and depression.

These clinical presentations were published in 1997 alongside works by many other professors and researchers in pharmacology and in the medical sciences, in a work that ran to more than 500 pages.[2] This work represented the first serious attempt to corroborate data from tradition and validate them with the most up-to-date science, with a view to a reevaluation of clinical practice. They capture the vision of tomorrow's medicine based on the concept of terrain and the scientific theory that underlies it: Endobiogeny.

We sent a copy of this book to all French medical journals. The only comment published in the medical press was this brief quip: "In this work you learn how to get rid of hiccups by chewing a sprig of tarragon ..."

Despite the absurdity of this rebuff, since that time, 20 years ago, many French and foreign doctors have been trained in the Endobiogenic approach. I have asked some of these colleagues, general practitioners, and specialists from various countries, England, United States, Mexico, Tunisia, and France to share their own findings and the results they have been able to observe in their patients. Here are some of their testimonies. This will provide a concrete illustration of the therapeutic outcomes of Clinical Phytotherapy, based on Endobiogenic principles, and may also give everyone the opportunity to read about cases that may concern them personally, or those close to them.

In the United States of America

The first testimony is that of Dr. Jean Bokelmann Professor of Medicine at the University in Pocatello, Idaho. She practices medicine in Idaho with her collaborators Laramie Wheeler DO[3] and Annette Davis CN[4] at the Endobiogenic Integrative Medical Center (EIMC).

"I first met Dr. Lapraz during the fall of 2004. He was leading a seminar in the EIMC[5] in Pocatello. In Endobiogeny he was presenting nothing less a new approach to medicine. I had been commissioned by the Idaho State University School of Medicine to present a residency program in integrative medicine to interns. This new medical approach has aroused considerable interest in the United States and has become very popular with patients. It aims to help them get the most out of natural plant-based treatments and promotes the wide use of vitamins, minerals, and dietary supplements. Another of its objectives is to find ways of reducing the side effects of chemical medicines. While this so-called integrative approach to medicine is gaining ground in America, and represents a small step toward reducing iatrogenic harm, it is very far from being a personalized and systematic model of human physiology.

I was immediately struck by the originality of the Endobiogenic approach. Working in France in close collaboration with medical colleagues, Drs. Christian Duraffourd and Jean-Claude Lapraz have developed a new clinical and scientific paradigm. They gave us a truly integrative vision of the physiological mechanisms at work in the human body. Their teaching expanded the concept of integrative medicine from the mere juxtaposition of various treatment methods, as is practiced in the United States into a new understanding of the real causes of disease and how to treat them.

Since 2004, in our center, we have successfully applied the principles of Endobiogeny to many common complaints, but also to serious pathological cases that have not been well served by conventional treatments. We have treated hundreds of patients suffering from all types of diseases with irrefutable success, regardless of the nature and the severity of their affection. Here are the five cases we have chosen to present.

First case: premenstrual syndrome and fatigue

This case concerns a young woman, aged 19, suffering from premenstrual syndrome, irregular periods, acne, fatigue, insomnia, and hair loss. The clinical examination and the analysis of the Biology of Functions reveal a certain number of dysfunctions. To give you some idea, we found an excessive activity of her alpha-sympathetic system, with a poor adrenal response; not only cortisol, but her estrogens, androgens, and progesterone all showed weak activity but, by contrast, her TRH activity and her insulin resistance were both high. We treated her with medicinal plants along Endobiogenic lines with a view to correcting those imbalances that had been identified. Her prescriptions included blackcurrant, Lady's mantle, salad burnet, lavender, bergamot, cinnamon, griffonia, and fabiana. After six months of treatment, we assessed her symptoms on a scale on which 0 scored complete failure, and 10 a complete success. She assigned a score between 8 and 9 for each of her complaints and declared herself to be now in perfect health, thanks to a treatment that permitted her to discontinue the numerous synthetic medicines she had taken previously.

Second case: hot flashes unresponsive to hormonal treatment

At the time of her first consultation at the EIMC center, this 55-year-old woman had been taking Levothyrox® for 6 years for thyroid deficiency. She had also undergone a complete hysterectomy with removal of her ovaries, and since then, had been prescribed synthetic estrogens, for persistent hot flashes, without success. She also takes tranquilizers for anxiety and insomnia.

After six months of Endobiogenic treatment, she recorded an improvement of her symptoms between 8 and 9 on the same scale. She was able to stop taking hormone replacement therapy altogether, which is unusual in women who have had their ovaries removed. We are now planning to gradually decrease her dose of Levothyrox®, monitoring her condition very carefully. This course of action is all the more justified now that modern medicine begins to worry about the potential for harm that long-term use of Levothyrox® poses for some patients.

Third case: epilepsy

This 39-year-old woman suffered from daily epileptic seizures for which she had taken potent synthetic medicinal products (Depakine, Trileptal) over a period of six months. She was being treated concurrently for thrombocytopenia, a blood disorder affecting her platelets. She also suffered from fatigue. The Endobiogenic examination showed an excessive alpha-sympathetic activity, a draining of her adrenal reserve, high levels of estrogen, and low levels of progesterone, together with severe ischemia (low tissue oxygen level) and a very low oxidation rate. The treatment with medicinal plants along Endobiogenic lines was directed towards correcting these various imbalances.

From the first month of treatment, she no longer had epileptic seizures every day; their frequency was reduced in about one per month. Her energy levels improved substantially, and her platelets were restored to normal levels. She discontinued the conventional medication in favor of the Endobiogenic treatment alone, and so avoided the potential unwanted effects of synthetic antiepileptic drugs, which can be very harmful.

Fourth case: depression

This young man, 19 years of age, came to see us complaining of depression, insomnia, acne, and gastrointestinal disorders. He had been treated with a succession of antidepressant drugs, Seroquel®, Pristia®, Prozac®, Trazadone®, none of which agreed with him at all.

After three months of Endobiogenic treatment, we asked him to assess the improvement of his symptoms, all of which he rated between

8 and 9 on the assessment scale. He was able to permanently discontinue any drug treatment.

Fifth case: degenerative disease of the nervous system

It is 3 years since we have embarked on treatment for this 70-year-old man, who suffered from multiple system atrophy (MSA), complicated by renal failure and generalized edema.

MSA is a very serious orphan neurodegenerative disease, for which there is currently no effective treatment. It develops into a major disability and is caused by progressive loss of neurons in several areas of the brain. The patient was bedridden and hospitalized at home, conventionally treated with morphine and Ativan (Lorazepam). His doctors gave him no more than a month to live.

We treated him with medicinal plants chosen according to Endobiogenic criteria, in conjunction with a low-protein diet and specific massage techniques with a view to reducing the inflammatory process. His strength and vitality rapidly improved. He was able to get about unaided and the hospitalization at home has been discontinued. For the past 3 years, he continues his background Endobiogenic therapy and his wife is able to provide the minimal care he needs."

Another testimony from the United States

Attention Deficit and Hyperactivity Disorder (ADHD) is a pressing issue these days, much discussed in the news, and continues to be a prevalent problem. Dr. Kamyar M. Hedayat,[6] a former pediatric critical doctor (Chicago, USA), presents the following case. In it, he recounts how he discovered Endobiogeny and applies it to the case of this child.

"As a pediatric specialist, I was trained in intensive care medicine at Stanford University and was involved in this specialty for 8 years in various private hospitals.[7] I was trained in understanding and treatment complex imbalances in physiology with the greatest technical advances and most powerful medications that American medicine places at our disposal. I came to believe that this system provided all I needed to know to treat children in the intensive care unit (ICU). I had spectacular results and import successes, saving many children's lives. Despite this, there were deep questions that challenged me. From the very beginning of my training in intensive care, I realized that there is no comprehensive theory or concept of health or illness. There was at that time an incomplete sense of the consequences of children surviving critical illnesses and their long-term development.

Also, I noticed that many children were what we called 'frequent fliers': they were repeatedly admitted with flare-ups of the same illness. I realized that our modern medicine does not actually treatment complex illnesses. In fact, I realized that our treatments often caused now illnesses to appear that didn't exist before.

I started studying various forms of 'integrative medicine' of the variety one finds taught in the US. Very quickly I realized that these approaches weren't very integrative at all. They taught the use of 'natural remedies' to simply replace pharmaceutical products and treat symptoms as they do.

But I knew from my training in pediatrics that each child is unique, and, moreover, it is different emotional, intellectual and physiological needs with each stage of development and phase of life. Sure, there were many natural tips and tricks I learned that reduced symptoms, but never did these various integrative approaches offer me a coherent explanation of why a specific child became ill, why each had differing symptoms with the same illness and why they required slightly different treatments. I kept asking myself in my medical practice, 'How can we treat a child at the root of their illness so that the illness doesn't return?'

When I learned that Dr. Lapraz was presenting a seminar on an integrative approach called Endobiogeny in the state of Idaho, I felt inspired to sign up for the course. I hoped that he could help me find the answers to my questions. Very quickly I perceived that Endobiogeny was the first contemporary medical model that could offer me scientific answers to my queries. I was at that time chief of intensive care and integrative medicine in Louisiana and required another doctor to care for my patients if I were to attend Dr. Lapraz's seminar. I approached the chief medical officer to arrange for this. Unfortunately, she was completely opposed to the idea simply because it was an integrative medicine conference. I stood up and quit my job on the spot without a second thought because I felt compelled to meet this man and learn about Endobiogeny. Fortunately, I found work in the ICU in Chicago.

Once I moved to Chicago, I had the good fortune of being able to continue my work in the ICU and to start a small private practice across the street from the hospital. Right away I started applying an

Endobiogenic approach both in the ICU and my private practice. Most of the children I treated in my practice were survivors of critical illness and the ICU. It was a new path that very few had dared to take on. In less than 2 years, I was so astonished and pleased with the results I had that I left ICU to dedicate myself full time to treating children and adults in outpatient practice only using the Endobiogenic approach.

According to the American Academy of Pediatrics, the pediatrician's role is to treat the 'child in their entirety, physiologic, mental, emotional, and social.' I could not conceive of a more complete approach to achieving this noble goal than Endobiogeny.

There were many interesting cases that I wanted to present. I chose two because I felt that they best illustrated the power of Endobiogeny to get to the root cause of illness and treat the whole child in a harmonious way based on who the person they are and not only the disease with which they were diagnosed.

First case: attention deficit hyperactivity disorder in a child

The first case is a 6-year-old boy with ADHD, emotional sensitivity and sensory integration disorder. This last condition is one in which a person is over- or under-sensitive to light, sound and/or touch. In his case, he was sensitive to the elastic in socks and the tags on underwear and wore neither. He was sensitive to certain textures and smells of foods. During meals, he fidgeted constantly to the great annoyance of his family.

The child's pediatrician rather summarily told the mother that all he could offer was a medication for ADHD. Otherwise, there were no treatments for his other symptoms. From my perspective, not only does the child suffer from such a condition, but so do his siblings, his parents, his friends and the learning environment at school. He was constantly shouting 'Don't do this!' 'Don't touch that!' and, 'Everyone stop what you're doing right now!' Unfortunately, he was frequently punished for these outbursts, which his family saw as an intentional attention-grabbing ploy.

He developed a reputation as a difficult child. His teachers considered him unintelligent due to his trouble paying attention. This constant struggle for control of him and rebellion against others resulted in a child with no respect for authority. In time, I feared, he would do serious harm to himself or others to gain attention.

The standard biomedical approach to this condition is to use a powerful mind-altering stimulant such as methylphenidate (Ritalin®), which increases dopamine levels in the brain.[8] These types of chemicals are not without dangers—they can result in hallucinations, migraine headaches, palpitations, loss of appetite with weight loss, convulsions, and a risk of drug addiction in adulthood.

These drugs suppress symptoms of ADHD. They do nothing to change the child's feeling that 'no one believes me, no one understands my suffering.' In fact, in can reinforce the feeling that 'they are trying to control me,' which is contrary to the human spirit of seeking freedom from control. The only goal of these synthetic products is to make the child uniform in a society that seeks conformity, no matter what the cost. The purpose of this type of treatment is not to seek the true cause of the disorder in order to serve the highest good of the child, his family and the society. In fact, it often results in a life of dependence on chemicals: amphetamines in the morning, anxiety medication in the afternoon, antidepressants and sedatives before bed ...

According to an Endobiogenic approach, the behavior of children diagnosed with ADHD is the consequence of the body trying to adapt itself to another fundamental problem. The root of the problem is rooted in a hypersensitive brain stem and an imbalance in the function of the adrenal gland. In fact, we have found that children with ADHD have too much attention. Their problem is that they see or hear or feel too much for their brains to process. As a result, they space out and shut down. In fact, fidgeting and moving is an attempt to fix the problem. When you tell an ADHD child to stop fidgeting, it's like telling a patient with high blood pressure to stop taking their medication. It should be the doctor's role to discover the heart of the matter, not just cover up symptoms so that Johnny can sit quietly in class and at the dinner table.

I started this boy exclusively on an Endobiogenic treatment without the use of stimulants. After eight weeks, his concentration improved and his hyperactivity was reduced according to his teachers, his parents, and himself. After he completed six months of treatment, his transformation was remarkable. He had become a boy who was able to sit and eat calmly with his family and hold excellent attention at school. He became a happy child with bright eyes—and a very happy mother!

How can we explain his improvements?

In his Biology of Functions (BoF), it appeared that the origin of his illness lay in the presence of multiple imbalances. First, he had trouble adapting to the energetic needs of his body. This was present at two levels. At the global hormonal level, he had insufficient adrenal function (low adrenal cortex index) and low sensitivity to thyroid hormones (low thyroid index). There was also a profound cellular insufficiency in making cell energy (elevated Proamyloid index) with a risk of improper cerebral development (elevated Amyloid index). This improved quite a bit after a few months of Endobiogenic treatment.

Glucose is a naturally occurring sugar used to make the currency of cellular energy called ATP. His body as a result of these deficiencies in delivering and using glucose for energy used certain compensatory mechanisms. The first was adrenaline. Adrenaline causes an intense and rapid rise in circulating blood sugar. This is helpful when your blood sugar levels are truly low, and you feel like fainting. In ADHD, blood sugar levels are often normal. The problem is how you use the sugar you have. Increasing blood sugar levels can cause the brain to feel hyper, or 'punch drunk.' The sudden rise in sugar drives certain brains to work harder and faster (incoherently), but not smarter. This results in trouble concentrating. Adrenaline also contracts muscle. This results in sudden or impulsive movements. As soon as adrenaline levels drop again, the ADHD brain feels starved for sugar because there is a sudden drop again. These children feel frustrated by their undependable use of sugar of energy. It's no wonder they exhibit disagreeable and even aggressive behavior at times.

This boy, like nearly all children we treat with ADHD, also had elevated levels of the neurohormone serotonin. In the brain, serotonin influences how quickly glucose enters the brain. Normally, if you have too much going in (after an adrenaline surge), your serotonin levels should drop to control the rate of entry. In ADHD children, this mechanism does not work well. Serotonin also increases how sensitive we are to textures, light, sound, and touch. The higher the serotonin levels in the brain, the more hypersensitive we become. This helps us understand another reason why ADHD kids show the types of behavior they do. They get easily overwhelmed by crowds or noisy environments, their stream of thought is disturbed by the smallest noise that the rest of us naturally tune out, and they seem to be picky about certain textures of foods or clothing or the seats the sit on.

In the BoF there is an index called the peripheral (i.e., body) serotonin level. Over 90% of total serotonin is actually in the gut, where it plays a role in digestion and absorption, especially of sugar. The lower the peripheral serotonin index is, the greater the brain serotonin tends to be. His peripheral serotonin index was very low—indicating that he had too much brain serotonin.

After about six months of an Endobiogenic treatment, his adrenal gland and thyroid function had both improved. As a result, he no longer needed to rely on excess adrenaline, so naturally his hyperactivity resolved. Parallel to his biological improvement was improvement in his behavior. The fact that some indexes did not return to normal indicated that he needed more extensive treatment to come to a good state of equilibrium.

Thanks to the judicious use of medicinal plants, carefully selected and personalized for each patient, my patients have experienced positive results repeatedly. All this without the need—in most cases—to use synthetic medications which could put patients at risk of side effects inherent to their use.

In summary, it seems quite clear that the abnormal behaviors and learning challenges that this boy with ADHD demonstrated were merely the consequence of underlying physiologic adaptations to trouble using sugar for energy. It was not an attention getting ploy or disrespect for authority because he was a bad apple in the bushel. When I explained to the boy and his parents that the origins of his behavior had a physiologic basis and was not malicious, they immediately understood that it was possible for him to change his life for the better.

Second case: a child with asthma

Asthma is a disorder that is common in childhood. Children with asthma can be considered fragile by some. They can be limited in their diet owing to certain foods that can trigger their asthma. They can be limited in their physical activity and their life in general. With the changing of the seasons, or after a rain, an asthma attack can come on and one can just hear the gasping for air and the wheezing in these little ones.

Naturally, during an asthma attack, the child must be treated with oxygen and powerful life-saving medications. We are not against the use of pharmaceuticals—only inappropriate selection, dosing or duration. Indeed, during an acute crisis, one must treat the child with fast acting drugs to combat the problem of lack of oxygen. Outside a crisis, an Endobiogenic approach can offer treatment of underlying issues that standard drugs cannot. That's not even to mention that recent studies show that long-term use of certain asthma medications actually increases the risk of dying from an asthma attack. Other studies show that they the bronchodilator and anti-inflammatory medications can lose their effectiveness over time.

In daily treatment, the standard-of-care approach is exclusively symptomatic and not without side effects like a racing heartbeat, shaky hands, a change in voice. In children, long-term use of steroids can slow down a child's rate of growth.

The Endobiogenic approach allows us to work with the terrain of the child with asthma. In modifying the imbalance at the origin of asthma, this approach gives the child and her parents hope in a future where the child may be free of drugs and still breath easily without fear of suffocating for air.

This case is about a 3-year-old little boy who suffered from a serious case of both asthma and eczema for 1 year when they came to my practice. He had been treated with steroids and other synthetic drugs during this 1 year, but his condition only continued to worsen. His dose of daily steroids was increasing, and he was using his rescue medications several times per month. I created a personalized Endobiogenic treatment using medicinal plants, probiotics, and omega-3 fatty acids. I also offered some advice in changing his diet and lifestyle based on his terrain in order to modify his sensitivity to external events and the internal reactions that would lead to an asthma attack.

After two months of treatment, his eczema completely disappeared— asthma and eczema share a common imbalance. After 1 year of Endobiogenic treatment, he no longer needed to use his long-acting puffer for asthma attacks (Salbutamol®) and reduced the dose of his everyday inhaled steroid. In the entire year, he only needed to use rescue steroids once. His immune system became much stronger as he had less viral colds and other common illnesses. This was important because infections can also be a cause of asthma attacks. His mother remarked to me that another child she knew with asthma, the same age as her son, continued to have worsening asthma over the last year. He was not treated Endobiogenically.

Asthma is a disease with a genetic basis. A realistic approach to asthma is to understand that it takes time to truly heal a child enough that they are no longer at risk of flare-ups. After 1 year, the child's terrain was still imbalanced but improved. At 2 years, it was stabilized.

While still not ideal, it was balanced enough that he no longer needed daily treatments and required steroids only once per year, not monthly. This demonstrates the importance of appreciating that treating the asthmatic child does not consist of a few tricks or quick fixes.

Endobiogeny is a thoughtful and rational system of treatment. It does not offer a magic pill that instantaneously cures a disease. It's a systematic approach to understand the true origin of disease. Endobiogeny is not opposed to the use of the drugs. The dictum of treatment is as follows: the power of the treatment should be in harmony with the degree of decompensation of the body. The weaker the patient has become, the more powerful the drug or dose of a plant-based treatment. The stronger the patient is, the less powerful the treatment needs to be.

Although I was not able completely stop the use of asthma medications altogether, I considered the Endobiogenic treatment a success for four reasons. Firstly, the number of the attacks of asthma was considerably reduced (down to once per year). Secondly, the child did not need hospitalization. Thirdly, the daily amount of steroids was reduced. Lastly, by also correcting the environmental, dietary and emotional issues related to asthma attacks, the mother and the child were able to better manage predilection to asthma—offering self-empowerment.

The Endobiogenic approach takes into account the true causes of disease. It has been a joy for me to offer this approach to help children find true health in all areas of their life: physical, emotional and mental. If more children can be treated Endobiogenically, the future of adult health may be profoundly altered."

Great Britain

I also asked the testimony of Colin Nicholls,[9] founder and president of the Endobiogenic Medicine Society (EMS), London. This is what he says:

"I first heard about Clinical Phytotherapy in the early 1980s, when I was living in Paris. On reading the *Cahiers de phytothérapie clinique* I was captivated by the new global approach that it proposed for treating patients and illness, and since then this has always been central to my own approach. After my return to the Great Britain I undertook the in-depth training required to become a 'medical herbalist,' a designation that is specifically British, but which also exists in Ireland and in countries with colonial links to Great Britain. 'Medical herbalists' are Phytotherapists who have the legal right in these countries to treat patients with medicinal plants.

Since the 1990s, people in the Great Britain who want to enter this profession have generally followed a university program that teaches them, together with the classical medical sciences, the pharmacological activities of plants and their traditional uses. In practice, while possessing a profound knowledge of classical Phytotherapy, medical herbalists use a wide range of therapeutic methods and diagnostic techniques, but they all claim to practice 'holistic or integrative medicine,' as it is termed in the United States.

I was passionate about the in-depth study of medicinal plants, but I felt there was a disjunction between this body of knowledge and the reductionist biochemical approach that characterized medical science teaching. The new and coherent global vision of pathophysiology, as provided by Endobiogeny, seemed to offer an answer to my questions. This is why, when I became editor of the newly launched *British Journal of Phytotherapy*, in the early 1990s, I got in touch with Dr. Lapraz and invited him and his colleagues to contribute a number of articles on Endobiogeny to the journal. Later, as lecturer in herbal medicine at Middlesex University, I invited Dr. Lapraz to give a series of seminars and workshops at the university—one or two a year—for medical herbalists in the Great Britain. On the strength of the interest aroused by this teaching, we created the EMS (becoming in 2017 the Endobiogenic Society) of which I am president. Over the years, a core group of practitioners has grown up around this training in Endobiogeny. They have all found that this original approach to illness has enabled them greatly to improve their results, especially in complex and difficult cases.

As an example, here are three cases treated by myself and my colleagues Paul Michael,[10] and Mara Baughman.[11]

First case: tonsillitis

This concerns a girl of 10, who was brought along by her mother because of repeated bouts of sore throat and tonsillitis that she had suffered since the age of 4. The attacks had become more and more frequent over the last two months or so. If the tonsillitis was not controlled with antibiotics, it quickly developed into otitis. The mother also said that her daughter had had bad breath since she was a toddler, and that this got worse during the crises, giving off an unpleasant 'fishy smell,' not only from her mouth but also from her vagina, and at the same time her anus became very itchy.

In general, the girl also suffered from a lot of catarrh, especially in the morning and in winter, as well as verrucas on the soles of her feet. On clinical examination, her hands and feet were cold and moist, her voice rather deep and husky, her pupils were enlarged, and her epigastric region was sensitive, especially on the right. This reflects a particular Endobiogenic imbalance that needed to be corrected.

The strategy adopted was to drain the liver and pancreas, to rebalance the intestinal flora, to reduce the overactivity of the parasympathetic and alpha-sympathetic nervous system, and to stimulate the immune system. For this we used green clay, essential oils and herbal tinctures, chosen for their ability to correct the observed imbalances. From the beginning of the treatment, which was simple and inexpensive, the girl experienced a progressive improvement in her respiratory symptoms and her bad breath. After four months, she had only had one slight sore throat, and, after seven months of treatment, she no longer had any infectious problem and her bad breath had completely disappeared.

Second case: chronic fatigue

A woman of 42 consulted because of chronic fatigue syndrome, which she had suffered from for about a year.

The trigger had been a streptococcal pharyngitis, following a long period of heavy stress. A fortnight after the sore throat started, she was assaulted by a reactive arthritis, with pains in her hips, fingers, and abdomen, together with a profound fatigue, almost liquid stools, insomnia, and a craving for sugar. From her medical history, one could see that she had suffered allergic-type episodes: she had had severe inflammatory reactions, with major facial swelling, after being stung by insects or exposed to flower or tree pollen. She had also suffered repeatedly from sinusitis and sore throat. At the consultation, she was so tired that she could barely speak; the least effort exhausted her and caused her to break out in a sweat. She had had to substantially reduce her hours of work. However, her mind was still very active, and she had difficulty relaxing. On examination, her hands and feet were very cold, suggestive of an overactive alpha-sympathetic.

A simple Biology of Functions, based on a full blood count, showed that the activity of her adrenal cortex, and of her circulating cortisol, was very low; by contrast, that of histamine—more than 100 times above the norm—reflected her increased allergic susceptibility.

The prescription included herbal tinctures chosen for their ability to correct the observed imbalances: i.e., that are antihistaminic and adaptogenic, support the adrenal cortex, curb the overactivity of the alpha-sympathetic and of histamine, decongest the pancreas, and modulate immune system activity. To reinforce the activity of the herbs, and with the same end in mind, we also advised the patient to cut out all sugar, to increase her water intake, and not to eat wheat-based foods for some time, in order to ease the pressure on her digestive system, and particularly on her pancreas.

Little by little, there was a progressive improvement in all her symptoms. After six months of treatment, and after some difficult episodes— hardly surprising in view of the difficulty of treating these types of symptoms, which often occur in a very degraded terrain—the patient was once again able to lead a completely normal life, without fatigue. She had gone back to work full time, was able to ride her bicycle, and no longer felt tired at the slightest effort. Besides this, her arthritis had disappeared, she was sleeping better, her digestion was good, and she no longer had any allergic reactions or respiratory problems. The results of her Biology of Functions, though they had improved, reflecting the normalization of her physical state, were still far from being entirely normal—which underlines the seriousness of the imbalance, and hence the ill-advisedness of interrupting the treatment too soon and the need to follow-up the patient over a long period of time in order to adapt the treatment plan to the development of her physical state.

Third case: ovarian cyst

This woman of 48, married without children, consulted in September, 2009, for an enormous cyst on the right ovary, 'as big as a large grapefruit,' which had first been discovered five months before, after the death of her father, to whom to she was very close.

An MRI scan also revealed the presence of bilateral endometrial tissue (or endometriosis) and a 6 centimeters pedunculated fibroid, which her gynecologist had been aware of for about 4 years. She had been advised to have her cystic right ovary removed, but she had preferred to try another approach.

At the first consultation, she appeared to be about 20 kilos overweight. She was a professional musician, and nearly every night, after the concert, she would go to a bar to have a drink with her colleagues. Her husband was suffering from an aggressive cancer that had just been diagnosed, and he had been told that he was in the terminal phase of his illness.

The prescription therefore considered all the imbalances that had been observed. Indeed, as Endobiogeny teaches us, the treatment must always be closely tailored to the individual patient and should never be a standardized treatment.

Using full-spectrum medicinal plant extracts, with a specific and precise action on the observed imbalances, the aim of the treatment in this case was to reduce estrogenic and especially androgenic activity, to reduce that of histamine and the alpha-sympathetic, to support the adrenal cortex, to rebalance thyroid activity, to reduce pelvic congestion, and, of course, to give dietary advice to complement the herbal treatment.

After seven months of treatment, in April, 2010, the cyst had shrunk in volume to the point where it was no longer visible on the MRI scan. The patient was in good form, despite the persistence of serious stress in her life. She had stopped drinking alcohol and had lost 16 kilos.

Given the result achieved—evident from the scan—and the remarkable progress that had been made—as shown by the indexes assessing growth (androgenic and growth indexes) and inflammation (indexes of inflammation, free radical nocivity, and potential histamine), we decided none the less to modify and adapt the treatment, because there remained a number of major imbalances to be corrected. Also, there was a risk that the severe psychological and emotional stress that she was undergoing would once again induce the biological imbalance, if she were left to herself with no corrective and maintenance treatment."

In Tunisia

This testimony is somewhat unusual because Dr. Najet Hajeri, who is a general practitioner in Tunis, presents her own case.

"I have been practicing as a family doctor in an inner-city district of Tunis since 1979. My practice took in the usual gamut of problems such as allergy, asthma, bowel disease, hypertension, and obesity and so I cared for many pediatric and geriatric patients, as well as obstetrics and gynecology. I had a leaning toward less aggressive, more natural treatments than those I had been taught in medical school on account of my own circumstances: about the time my second child was born some 6 years ago, I developed a painful elephantiasis[12] in my right leg. Neither the phlebotomists nor the cardiologists managed to do anything to alleviate the considerable pain and smarting that never left me. It was in 1988 that I first came across homeopathy, and began a course of homeopathic treatment, which gave me relief and gradually, in a few months, the edema slowly reduced, and my leg regained its shape.

Having seen the benefits in my own case, I started to prescribe homeopathic treatments for my patients. I found natural treatments to be effective at reducing the frequency of recurrent upper respiratory disorders, psychosomatic digestive problems, skin allergies, and so on. I also stopped prescribing corticosteroids, which spoiled the quality of life for my patients through their adverse effects. But I was not completely satisfied with the results obtained with homeopathy and I was looking for a more comprehensive approach. At much the same time I became aware of the extent of the menopausal and peri-menopausal complaints suffered by my female patients. Indeed, women began to refuse the hormone replacement therapies prescribed by my gynecology colleagues. A pharmacist friend told me about the courses in Endobiogenic Phytotherapy taught by French doctors at the Faculty of Pharmacy of Monastir and, in 1991, I decided to enroll on this program. I found explanations and answers to the many questions that confronted me every day about the chronic disorders, which homeopathy had been unable to resolve completely.

I started by taking care of my own peri-menopausal state which had caused me to gain a few kilos, to have premenstrual irritability and hot flashes. Most importantly, it coincided with the appearance of diabetes with my blood glucose hovering between 1.5 g and 1.70 g. I had not managed to reduce my dietary carbohydrates and I had an intense sugar craving. After the first three months of plant-based treatment, established according to Endobiogenic rules, I was able to gradually change my eating habits and from the second month of treatment my blood glucose quickly normalized. I was also prone to recurrent bouts of nasopharyngitis, which would begin in the early days of fall. They had become less frequent with homeopathic treatment, but with Phytotherapy they completely disappeared.

Returning to my patients and how they got on, the Endobiogenic approach allowed me to obtain the following results:

- Diabetic patients obtained better control of their blood glucose, which allowed me to reduce their allopathic treatment. They also had fewer reactions to the change of seasons.
- Patient presenting with a range of common problems, such as osteo-arthritis, early benign prostatic hyperplasia, bowel disorders, and many other problems, reported an improvement of almost 70% in their symptoms after three months of treatment.
- Cardiac patients, with stents, and following bypass surgery and other serious problems also reported a significant improvement after taking Endobiogenic treatment. Witnessing these results their cardiologists encouraged them to continue on the plant-based therapy, even if they personally knew nothing about this method of treatment.
- Women with large uterine fibroids, who were being considered for hysterectomy, saw their menstrual cycle become regular, their periods becoming lighter, with significantly reduced pelvic pain. They were able to sail through the menopause, without the need to remove their fibroids, which no longer caused them any problems.
- In the case of children suffering from asthma, allergic rhinitis, and all the other usual respiratory problems, their pediatricians could not fail to notice the efficacy of terrain Phytotherapy. I treat many my colleagues and their children.

Since 2005, when I moved my medical practice to central Tunis, I restructured my consultations based on the one to two hours I devote to the examination of each patient, so that I can get a deeper understanding of their terrain. Patients understand the reasons for this change and they appreciate it, because they realize that integrative medicine needs time to help them better understand their conditions and to take responsibility for their own care in an informed and responsible manner. I continue to take professional development courses in Endobiogeny and Clinical Phytotherapy in Paris, just as a new biological approach was born: the Biology of Functions. This method opens up promising horizons for clinical assessment, and will help us interpret, clarify and quantify the conclusions we draw from the consultation and examination of the patient."

In Mexico

Clinical Phytotherapy based on Endobiogeny knows no frontiers, and produces the same positive effects regardless of wherever on the planet it is practiced, corroborated by the following testimony of Dr. Paul Hersch,[13] from Mexico City:

"Mexico is characterized by considerable cultural diversity, with a rich knowledge of 'herbalist medicine.' Different strands of medical knowledge were happily married with an abundance of mainly plant resources, and in current use in naturopathy and traditional medicine. Thanks to this convergence of differing, but complementary approaches, original medical research into public health was instigated in Mexico City. Developed within the framework of the Integrative Medicine Program of the Ministry of Health of the Federal District, (i.e., within the public health service of the nation's capital, its principal aim was the fostering of the medicinal use of plants).[14]

To launch this project, several institutions worked collaboratively with the Department of Health: *Sociedad Mexicana de Fitoterapia Clínica* (SMFC) (The Society of Clinical Phytotherapy in Mexico), The International Society of Endobiogenic Medicine and Integrative Physiology (SIMEPI) and the National Institute of Anthropology and History through its research program 'Social Agents of the Medicinal Flora of Mexico.'

From September, 2009, thanks to the collaboration of these organizations, a teaching program in Clinical Phytotherapy was set up, based on Endobiogeny. This is a dynamic approach to physiology that offers a rigorous and integrative methodology allowing for the scientific use of medicinal plants in medical practice, beyond their purely empirical and symptomatic use. The aim was to train 45 doctors practicing in Mexico City in Clinical Phytotherapy. Most of the clinical training was conducted by members of SIMEPI, namely Doctors Jean-Claude Lapraz, Jean-Christophe Charrié, Alain Carillon, and Kamyar Hedayat. By July, 2011, having finished the course, a series of seminars of one week per month, spread over 18 months, the doctors began to integrate Clinical Phytotherapy into their practices.

In September of that same year, the *Centro De Especialidades Medicas Integrales* (CEMI) was launched in Mexico City, in the presence of the Minister of Health and the City's Mayor. This specialist center is a hub for the Integrative Medicine Program (IMP) that draws on a network of public health medical centers spread throughout the vast city. This adoption of Clinical Phytotherapy by the public health system of such an important capital as Mexico City, favors the integration of the remarkable body of Mexican herbal knowledge and materia medica into mainstream medicine. This has important implications for the economy and for the preservation of cultural identity and, perhaps more importantly, will contribute to greater efficacy and an enhanced quality in the delivery of medical.

Doctors Paul Hersch, Miguel Poujol,[15] and Ana Sanchez[16] (CEMI Center) have chosen the following case histories from among the many patients treated in Mexico based on the Endobiogenic approach.

First case: risk of sterility

This 28-year-old woman underwent surgical removal of a cyst on her right ovary on March 13, 2009. On April 10, 2009, very soon after the operation, a large cyst of 27 cubic centimeters was discovered on her left ovary, so it seemed that as if she had succumbed to a polycystic ovarian syndrome in a very short time. She came to consult with us at our center on April 16, 2009, because her surgeon had advised her to undergo further surgical intervention but she preferred to give plant-based treatment a try before considering further surgery. She was at a loss to understand how the disease could have spread so quickly to her remaining ovary.

The Endobiogenic evaluation showed strong alpha-sympathetic tone with a delayed beta-sympathetic response, very severe pelvic congestion, adrenal insufficiency, high overall estrogenic and androgenic activity with progesterone insufficiency, and hepatic and intestinal congestion. The treatment, prescribed according to the Endobiogenic approach, included vitex (*Vitex agnus castus*) to slow down estrogens and gonadotrophins, plantain (*Plantago major*) to ensure hepato-renal drainage, and cajuput and lavender for their anti-infective action on the reproductive system and to relieve pelvic congestion, and regulate her autonomic nervous system. These medicinal plants were combined with sedative other plants such as motherwort and lemon balm, and with blackcurrant and yarrow to support her progesterone.

After following this treatment for three months, the ovarian cysts completely disappeared, and the ultrasound showed her ovaries to be entirely normal. The scheduled surgical procedure was canceled.

Second case: hyperthyroidism

A 57-year-old woman came to us to consult about her hyperthyroidism, which had been diagnosed three months earlier. As soon as the diagnosis had been made, she was prescribed a daily dose of Atenolol (a beta blocker) and three tablets of Tapazol (an anti-thyroid medicinal product). In spite of taking these very potent drugs, which were designed to block her thyroid, she nonetheless continued to suffer from tachycardia and tremors.

Taking an Endobiogenic approach allowed us to identify a serious abnormality in the functioning of her autonomic nervous system: a very strong alpha-sympathetic and beta-sympathetic system, pointing to the role that stress played in triggering her illness. Additional evidence for the importance of stress was provided by the very high level of the TRH index that denoted excessive peripheral and central thyroid activity. This index implied that the events that triggered her illness were strongly emotional in nature. Our interview with the patient confirmed this to be the case. Unsurprisingly, we found a very strong histamine activity and a high level of cortisol, which all went to show that she was in the throes of a very strong adaptive response to the difficulties she was going through in her personal life. Her pancreas reacted strongly as might be expected to all this turmoil and so we saw a very high activity of her insulin, contributing further to dysregulation and imbalance. Her ovaries had obviously been affected by this pathological sequence, and the index that evaluated their activity showed a fall in her estrogen levels with an excess of androgens.

We put in place a precise treatment plan to correct all these imbalances, using plantain for its antihistamine activity, sage to support her estrogens, hawthorn to slow down the beta and alpha-sympathetic activity and reduce tachycardia, lavender to further slow down alpha-sympathetic activity, gypsywort and *Fabiana* to slow down the thyroid at the central level, and turnip to slow it down in the periphery.

After following this treatment for a month, she was able to stop taking Atenolol. Eight months later, she was only on half a tablet of Tapazol a day. The tremor had disappeared and her pulse rate had normalized.

Third case: food poisoning

Before she came to see us, this 46-year-old woman had been hospitalized with food poisoning over a period of three months for which she had needed rehydration and high-dose antibiotic therapy. Since then, she has suffered from permanent diarrhea, despite two additional courses of antibiotics (Ciprofloxacin). The stool tests show no evidence of parasites.

The Endobiogenic evaluation of this patient shows that she has an overactive parasympathetic system with a reactive alpha-sympathetic, severe liver and pelvic congestion, and major intestinal dysbiosis.

To correct these imbalances, we prescribed her peony to reduce her intestinal spasms, walnut for its astringent action on the digestive tract, and cuachalalate for its astringent and anti-inflammatory action on the digestive tract. This plant (*Amphipterygium adstringens*) is extensively used in Mexico, with excellent results. We also gave her essential oils of lavender and thyme for their anti-infective action and to regulate the autonomous nervous system. As well as an infusion of guava for her to drink for three days, we put her on a seven-day course of green clay (mainly *illite*), rich in mineral substances, which very actively adsorb the microorganisms and their toxins. We also prescribed probiotics for two weeks.

In less than ten days, she was cured: her three months of severe digestive disorders (despite multiple courses of antibiotics) had completely disappeared.

Fourth case: dry cough

This little boy, aged 7, is acutely sensitive to the cold and to cold foods. He had suffered for nearly 14 months from a continuous dry cough, which had been treated without success by numerous courses of antibiotics, antihistamines, and cortisone. His overall condition is poor. He does not sleep at all well and has nightmares. He is easily distracted, has great difficulty with attention in school and his behavior creates a lot of problems with other children. His clinical examination and Endobiogenic assessment show a significant neurovegetative imbalance with an excess of histamine, which induces respiratory hyper-reactivity. His hyperinsulinism will tend to inflammation and consequent congestion of the airways thus increasing their susceptibility to infection. He is prescribed dietary measures to relieve the activity of the pancreas, and the mother is advised to reduce his intake of sweets and dairy products. His prescription includes plants for correcting the imbalance of the child's terrain: limeflowers, passionflower, essential oil of lavender, and *Cordia morelosana*, a Mexican plant with anti-infective properties which is traditionally recommended for throat and lung problems and in whooping cough. Additionally, Magnesium is prescribed for its ability to help maintain general equilibrium.

After following this simple and inexpensive treatment for a month his cough disappeared and all his other symptoms improved considerably. The child's behavior in school is no longer a cause for complaint. He is no longer irritable and his sleep and dreams are quite normal. He can now go out in cold weather without impunity, and he was even able to eat ice cream without coughing, which, of course, he should not continue to do, knowing the important role sugar plays in the genesis and maintenance of respiratory infections.

Fifth case: respiratory allergy

This young girl, 7 years old, has suffered respiratory allergies for more than a year, with recurrent bouts of coughing. The immunotherapy given to her against dust mites and cockroaches has offered her no relief. She is on a permanent drug regime of Montelukast (a leukotriene receptor antagonist), Rinelon (anti-allergic), and, from time to time, corticosteroids. Her Endobiogenic examination revealed her to be in a state of vagotonia, with an excess of histamine. Her adrenal glands responded poorly to the excessive output of the stress hormone ACTH. She was hyperinsulinic and both her liver and pancreas were very congested. We set about formulating a treatment plan that would address all these disturbances. We advised her to greatly reduce her consumption of dairy products and sugar, to replace the wheat flour with corn, to stop snacking, and avoid heavy meals in the evening. The prescription itself was simple: plant-based digestive enzymes (papain) before each meal for a month, and two plant-based medicines. The first was a mixture of essential oils (lavender and thyme) in mother tinctures of plantain and hawthorn, 50 drops to be taken morning and evening. The second was a glycerin macerate of blackcurrant buds, 60 drops to be taken also morning and evening.

After following this course of treatment for one month, this little girl stopped having respiratory tract infections, and within a few weeks experienced a 90% improvement in all her symptoms, which allowed her to discontinue all her chemical medication."

In France

Doctors in our country have devoted themselves for many years to the practice of Endobiogeny and to the development of this comprehensive approach to clinical medicine. Dr. Jean-Christophe Charrié, general practitioner, gives the following personal account.

"During my second year of medicine, I met by chance Dr. Christian Duraffourd, and then Dr. Jean-Claude Lapraz. From the outset, I felt deeply drawn to their approach to the sick and their way of listening, to their holistic respect for man and nature and the fact that they placed the patient at the center of their care. Very quickly, I wanted to learn from them, but their response was always the same: 'first finish your medical studies and only after that, will you be able to start training in Clinical Phytotherapy and Endobiogeny.' Frustrated and rebellious, as one can be at this age, I was much at odds with the conventional training in which I was engaged. I felt restricted by a system that tried to force complex questions into a multiple-choice format where only single answers can be given and then are marked by a computer. My opposition landed me in quite a lot of trouble, before I understood the need to buckle down and conform to the system. Eventually, in 1998, I presented my thesis, for which I was awarded a national first prize, conferred by the Faculty of Medicine Xavier-Bichat. Looking back, and currently practicing Endobiogeny, I realize they had been right. My practice is based on the core principles of the art of medicine, but embodies also the concept of integration, which leads to a broader understanding of the mechanisms at work in living organisms. Endobiogeny brings with it a truly humanist dimension, putting Louis Pasteur in his rightful place, and giving the clinical practice of Claude Bernard the value it should have never lost. Therefore, I dutifully completed my studies before embarking on my training in Clinical Phytotherapy, which I received in Monastir, Tunisia, from 1997 to 2000.

Why Tunisia? Simply because the Tunisians have understood, well before the French, the need to reintegrate the use of medicinal plants into their healthcare system, with the condition that they be prescribed by doctors and prepared by pharmacists. As Doctors Christian Duraffourd and Jean-Claude Lapraz were the recognized authorities on the medical use of medicinal plants, Professor Chemli invited them to lead this clinical Department. They taught there for over 10 years until 2004, when the program was discontinued for reasons that had nothing to do with medical science, but everything to do with local politics.

For 11 years, I practiced medicine part-time at the Hospital of La Rochelle, where I implemented a care system[17] ensuring effective support of chronic wounds in the Dermatology Department, and the outpatient follow-up. The integrative vision of the human being, obtained thanks to Endobiogeny, helped me establish personalized treatments using natural-based products (medicinal plants, clay, etc.) for patients suffering from skin diseases. I had the opportunity to use them on many occasions in the treatment of wounds, often with impressive results.[18,19]

My work was based on results obtained within the framework of humanitarian outreach schemes that were conducted by Dr. Lapraz in five West African countries through the auspices of The Raoul Follereau Foundation between 1994 and 1997. They were concerned with the treatment of perforating plantar ulcers in patients suffering from leprosy, lesions that would often lead to the amputation of part of the affected limb. The report of Dr. Abdoulaye Ndiaye, who was the first advisor to the Minister of Health of Senegal, provided ample evidence for the superior healing action of illite green clay on these lesions, compared with conventional antiseptic treatments.[20] Most regrettably, these programs have not been continued.

I also took part, along with Dr. J. C. Lapraz, Dr. A. Carillon, and others, in the implementation of a large humanitarian project in Madagascar. Its aim was to help control the cholera epidemic of 1999–2000 by the use of a certain type of green clay. The results of the randomized controlled trial of the green clay/illite protocol against conventional care were presented in May, 2000, by Dr. R. Robinson, doctor at the Department of Communicable Disease Surveillance, Department of Epidemiological Surveillance at the Third International Conference of Clinical Phytotherapy held in Monastir (Tunisia) organized under the aegis of the Minister of Health and Scientific Research. The results showed that a favorable outcome of clinical signs of cholera is achieved much more quickly when illite is combined with conventional therapy. This means that vomiting stopped sooner and dehydration was drastically reduced, both of which are crucial for a better prognosis. The average duration of a hospital stay is reduced with illite clay, and the overall mortality rate is lower than with conventional treatment alone.

My professional life was otherwise devoted to private medical practice and the unceasing pursuit of learning. The choice I made to practice 'clinical medicine,' concerned more with the outcome for each patient taken as a unique individual, rather than 'evidence-based medicine' with its imposition of standard treatments, was not an easy choice to make. Indeed, this kind of practice involves a great deal of time spent with the sick. We can expect to devote a minimum of one hour to every consultation. As the current practice in France requires doctors to devote, on average, fewer than ten minutes per patient, such a choice means that the physician cannot be covered by the health system. As a result, the doctor cannot sign a covenant with the Department of Social Security, and so loses out to colleagues who do. As well a loss of income for the doctor who makes this choice, the patient also incurs a cost, as their medical consultation will not covered under the National Health System. But that is the price of freedom, such as it is in our country.

Neither I, nor any of my patients have ever regretted this choice because the benefits have exceeded all our expectations. Yes, you are satisfied with the choice you made when a woman suffering from very severe ankylosing spondylitis, who had struggled in to the first appointment on walking sticks, returns six months later walking normally. She reports that her quality of life has improved enormously thanks to her treatment by medicinal plants, rather than the many molecules prescribed by specialists over the years. Of course, you are satisfied with your choice when a young woman suffering from a genetic disease that made her lungs fragile and condemned her to courses of antibiotics every month. Exhausted and with her survival put at 2 years at best, is in excellent shape 5 years later with plenty of plans for the future and has to take only one or two short courses of antibiotics per year, thanks to her Endobiogenic treatment. Yes, you are happy with the choice you made when a 6-year-old child with severe chronic asthma, and whose heavy cortisone regimens has impaired his growth, is now growing normally and in much better general health; in less than a year of Endobiogenic treatment, all chemical medication is stopped and he only takes medicinal plants as background therapy.

All the physicians who practice Endobiogeny and use medicinal plants in their practice can tell similar stories. If only there were many more of us! If only we could be given the opportunity to present this knowledge to the French faculties of medicine! There is no doubt that the health of our children, and ours too, would be substantially improved.

An opportunity appeared elsewhere: the Parliamentary Assembly of the Federal District of Mexico City voted in 2009 for a law requiring the free public health system of this large city to include medicinal plants. This would require the training of Mexicans physicians, so when asked to join this project, I did not hesitate for a moment. This was the first venture in the world to respond to a call from the WHO. In order to be fully involved in its implementation, I had to resign from my hospital post."

Dr. Alain Carillon likewise shares his thoughts.

"As a general practitioner, 'lynchpins of the health system,' I was trained by eminent specialists outstanding in their respective fields. I completed a number of internships in different hospital departments and I so saw at first hand the how certain diseases could bring gravely ill people into hospital.

I was, therefore, greatly surprised when I set up in practice as a general practitioner from my very first patient. None of the symptoms bore any resemblance to the diagnostic and therapeutic criteria I had assimilated during the long course of my studies. Except for a few emergencies, the great majority of diseases are not of the same type or the same severity as those encountered in hospital practice. How, then, to address these common and, in most instances, benign pathologies? What kind of treatment should I prescribe? Should I just do as I did in the hospital? And what should I do with cases that continually relapse?

Another problem that concerned me was how to establish the best outcomes for patients in the long-term, as I came to realize that current official guidelines for conventional treatment are likely to have far more disadvantages than benefits for the patient in the long run.

The Endobiogenic approach with its careful and comprehensive physiological evaluation of each patient began, little by little, to answer these questions, one at a time. These clinical tools that Drs. Duraffourd and Lapraz and their coworkers had developed, were backed up by over 30 years of daily clinical practice.

Florence's case

This is a good example of a case that might have turned out very differently had she not been assessed by an integrative approach, which tried to find the physiological meaning of the various diseases that had afflicted her throughout her life. Her medical history is as follows:

- At the age of 35, she underwent surgery for mitral valve stenosis, because of an acute rheumatic fever that she acquired at the age of 6.
- After the age of 40, several crises of biliary colic, with many stones in her gallbladder.
- She reached menopause at the age of 48, when she was put on hormone replacement therapy.

- At the age of 52, she fractured her ankle, for which she needed a cast, which led to local bone-loss.
- At the age of 52, after very suddenly developing cardiac arrhythmia, she suffered a cerebral embolism with paralysis of the hand that gradually resolved. She was put on anticoagulants and given antiarrhythmic medication: Serecor® (hydroquinidine) and Cordarone®.
- At the age of 53, onset of osteoporosis, and hypertension with a systolic pressure of 220, for which she was given hypotensive medication (Prestol®). She was found to have severe hypercholesterolemia,[21] which required the discontinuation of her hormonal treatment and the prescription of a hypolipidemic drug (Zocor®).

First consultation

She was 55 when she first came to see me. I devised a personalized plant-based treatment for her that aimed to reduce her blood pressure and her blood lipids, as well as her high alpha-sympathetic nervous system; the plan was to help her remineralize, while at the same time lending support to her gonadal and thyroid axes. She was to take these treatments alongside all the drugs that had been prescribed by her other doctors.

Second consultation (after four months)

I wrote to her cardiologist to explain that I had made a full and comprehensive evaluation of her hormonal state, taking all her endocrine axes into account in an integrative manner and noting their clinical and biological development. Given all this and her postmenopausal state, I felt that there was a high probability that the Cordarone[22] she was currently taking might well cause her to develop hypothyroidism. I suggested that he might prescribe an alternative antiarrhythmic drug that would not interfere with her endocrine equilibrium. In his reply, the cardiologist admitted the potential risk, but insisted that the latter could easily be controlled by another drug. He added that, in his opinion, her hypercholesterolemia had nothing to do with her endocrine equilibrium and insisted that she continue taking the prescribed hypolipidemic medication. He does not consider my concern to be justified.

Taking full account of the positive results, both clinical and biological, obtained during these first four months of Endobiogenic treatment, I advised the patient to steadily reduce her dose of both the hypolipidemic and the anti-hypertensive drugs and to continue taking the plant-based course of treatment concurrently.

Third consultation (after seven months)

The patient tells me that she had been hospitalized with a biliary crisis, and was rushed into an emergency operation to remove her gallbladder, during which she developed pericarditis and then went into atrial fibrillation, despite being on antiarrhythmic medication. In the course of this consultation, I make some specific adjustments to her plant-based treatment and, based on her clinical and biological results, which had normalized, I decided to stop the hypolipidemic (Zocor®), and hypotensive (Prestol®) drugs, as well as the calcium and vitamin D but to maintain, of course, the antiarrhythmic and anticoagulant drugs (Serecor® and Cordarone®).

Regular follow-up consultations

I monitor her state very closely, especially her thyroid status. I note that her clinical and biological condition has stabilized well as she continues with the complementary plant-based treatment. This consists of plants with alpha-sympatholytic, antispasmodic, and hypotensive properties; others reduce blood lipids and inhibit aggregation of platelets. Other plants help her gonadal axis initiate metabolic demand which must be accommodated especially by her thyroid axis that has been disrupted by the iodine overload induced by Cordarone®.

I assess her biological state regularly with particular emphasis on her thyroid keeping a close eye on developments so as to modify her treatment towards normalizing her Endobiogenic state. She continues to take Cordarone®, as she still has severe arrhythmia in spite of having electrical cardioversion at various times. Her drug treatment is failing to reduce her tachyarrhythmia, but she has to continue the treatment on the advice of her cardiologist, who has now decided to stop the Serecor®.

Two years and three months after the first consultation

The patient is taking medicinal plants alone for her blood cholesterol and hypertension and I note that both these have now been brought into normal range, but the patient is still suffering from severe arrhythmia.

Her biological assessment reveals a new development: a slightly overactive thyroid[23] that paradoxically conceals an underlying underactive state. The thyroid axis has reacted to an underlying peripheral insufficiency by making an upward jump and may presage a move towards Graves' disease.

Consequently, I wrote again to her cardiologist pointing out the significant risk of Graves' disease (hyperthyroidism)[24] and he then agrees to stop the Cordarone®. The plant-based treatment had maintained this patient in a state of relative equilibrium for over 2 years, in spite of the Cordarone®. While it may be indicated for heart conditions it was contraindicated in her case because of her hormonal disposition.

Two years and four and a half months after the first consultation

The patient declares that she does not feel at all well. I see her as an emergency, and she is physically unrecognizable, presenting all the characteristic signs of a sudden and severe onset of textbook hypothyroidism.[25]

The cardiologist is concerned that if she were to remain in such an extreme hypothyroid state, she runs a major risk of cardiac decompensation. He is worried that if she is prescribed thyroid hormones, they 'will probably trigger cardiac problems,' so he decides to refer her to an endocrinologist, who in turn does not know what to do.

Subsequent consultations

The patient and I decide to keep in regular contact by telephone between consultations and for her to have frequent biological tests. Relying exclusively on plant-based treatments, and without any additional replacement therapy, we were able to report a rapid reduction in the clinical signs of hypothyroidism and other biological problems. This was corroborated by blood tests, which showed a steady decrease of thyroid stimulating hormone, and within a few months, her peripheral thyroid hormones were all within the normal range. Her treatment involved stimulating her thyroid with non-iodine remedies such as ginger, Chinese boxthorn (*Lyceum barbarum*) and oats; an immunomodulator (*Robinia pseudoacacia*); cardio-tonic and cardio-regulatory plants (lily of the valley, hawthorn, lemon balm, lavender), along with other plants to support her gonadic and adrenocorticotropic axes.

Twenty years later

The patient has been monitored regularly and now her occasional bouts of arrhythmia are clinically insignificant, without any attendant cardiovascular problems. Her blood pressure is normal as are her blood lipids, with lowered risk of atheromatous disease, osteoporosis, or osteoarthritis. Her endocrine system is in equilibrium: she has suffered no relapse of hypothyroidism and did not even test positive for thyroid-specific antibodies. Her digestion is good and problem-free. All this balance was achieved with plant-based treatments, based on an integrative Endobiogenic approach, in conjunction with the conventional anticoagulant drug (Préviscan®) that we decided to maintain. All other synthetic medicinal drugs were discontinued.

This example, which describes over 20 years of treating this patient and monitoring her progress, is by no means atypical and represents the very real possibilities on offer to patients by the Endobiogenic approach which allows for problems to be anticipated and thereby prevented. Drug treatments can sometimes provoke serious decompensation when they focus exclusively on symptoms. They can also precipitate pathologies that might have been foreseen, thyroid problems in this example, which the conventional approach tends not to take into account. Far from being guesswork, this approach is based on an integrative Endobiogenic assessment, which is both rigorous and accurate, and takes into account both the clinical and the biological state. Is this not genuine preventative medicine?

Endobiogeny also offers the possibility that conventional drug treatments may, in the medium- or long-term, be discontinued. These drugs are often very powerful and yet they are generally to be taken for life. Of course, any discontinuation would be absolutely conditional on understanding that the symptoms and the disease are manifestations of underlying particular to that patient. Resolving the imbalances that induced the pathology in the first place is the avowed aim of Endobiogeny. Is this not a real patient-oriented medical approach?

In the end, does this not illustrate that with this approach to health it is possible to combine high-class medical care with budgetary savings, which will be of benefit both to the individual and to society?"

By way of conclusion, here is the testimony of a dermatologist, Dr. Nicole Guiot Tabernat who is based in Paris.

"After several years of practicing dermatology, I had the opportunity to meet Dr. Lapraz and collaborate with him on some cases that were resistant to conventional therapies.

Eighteen months previously, Dr. Lapraz and I had embarked on a research project (which is ongoing) on 38 patients (20 women and 18 men), all suffering from psoriasis, some of them for over 20 years. Psoriasis is a chronic skin condition for which the causes have not been fully established by modern medicine. It is a scaly, often very itchy condition that affects nearly 4% of the French population. The lesions consist of dry red or pinkish patches covered with white scales, and tend to affect the elbows, arms and hands, lower legs and feet, as well as the scalp.

Patients with psoriasis often experience significant relationship problems because of their unsightly lesions, which often shed copious amounts of dry skin. Currently, there is no cure for this affliction, and conventional treatments offer only temporary relief. Dermatologists sometimes have to prescribe powerful therapies such as immunosuppressive drugs such as Cyclosporine, and antimetabolites such as Methotrexate, or biotherapies. All of these have potentially severe side effects and so requiring a close monitoring of the patient's liver.

Our research objective has been to elucidate the Endobiogenic imbalances that may underlie this type of skin disease. Our initial findings, which are in the process of verification, have used the Biology of Functions to demonstrate the important role played by the adrenocorticotropic hormonal axis with a very active alpha-sympathetic system, both involved in the stress response, together with high levels of ACTH and histamine. Our findings also show that other hormonal systems are involved, in particular a very high estrogen activity of in bodily tissues activated by FSH, its central controller. We found that insulin, a hormone secreted by the pancreas, and which plays an important role in cellular nutrition is also implicated in psoriasis.

While these functional abnormalities have been found in all the patients in the study, nonetheless, each of them possesses an individual Endobiogenic profile. These variations allow for a better understanding of the different presentations of the disease: psoriasis associated with severe inflammation, or on the contrary without inflammation, presence or absence of itch, or of pustules. Whether the spread of the disease was generalized or localized and even the specific location of lesions was explained by the role played by each of the hormonal mechanisms involved. These findings offer the obvious advantage that the treatment can be targeted in a precise manner towards the correction of the underlying state that is the root cause of the disease rather than the elimination of the disease itself.

Current medical research tends to be focused on the identification of genetic determinants of susceptibility and on the analysis of functional changes made in skin cells by T lymphocytes in order to develop more selective immunosuppressant drugs. As important as an understanding of such phenomena may be, it essentially addresses the disease only in its relationship with the skin but fails to take account of how the skin functions in its relationship with the other organs and their various regulatory functions. This is why we believe that a more comprehensive approach to psoriasis should be envisioned, one that would expand our understanding of this disease with a view to finding truly integrative ways of managing it.

When used according to specific rules, the medicinal plants present a real hope for patients suffering from psoriasis, as we will shortly see from the following two examples. They are quite different patients, each of whom has been suffering from psoriasis for many years. They are chosen from among other similar cases, and they will exemplify a view of psoriasis taken not as an isolated phenomenon, but rather as a sign of a global imbalance in the body of the sufferer.

First case: generalized psoriasis

Born in 1949, this man has suffered from generalized psoriasis for over 12 years. I have been treating him for over 9 years using various local and systemic treatments, but have not resorted to giving him the most up-to-date molecular biotherapy on account of their potential for severe side effects.

In this case, following an in-depth analysis by Dr. Lapraz, a course of Phytotherapy was initiated based on the Endobiogenic approach with the aim of rebalancing the patient in his entirety, to calm his sympathetic system, to stimulate the activity of his adrenal glands, to slow down his thyroid and to ensure hepatic drainage. After nine months of treatment, not only have the psoriatic lesions completely disappeared but the patient now also enjoys a restful night's sleep and no longer wakes tired in the morning.

Second case: localized psoriasis

This woman, born in 1955, has had psoriasis for about 20 years, mainly on her feet. She has undergone numerous conventional courses of treatment. As in the case of the previous patient, following a course of

Phytotherapy, her psoriasis has completely vanished and, currently, she continues to have a perfectly healthy skin. The Phytotherapy treatment she was prescribed included plants with anti-thyroid properties as well as drainage of her liver and pancreas.

So, while conventional topical therapies successfully produce an immediate improvement, Endobiogenic therapy helps prevent the disease from recurring and, furthermore, improves the patient's overall health by taking into account the person's terrain and by investigating the root causes that lie behind the symptoms."

In conclusion: why sacrifice medicinal plants?

As we have just seen, the therapeutic success obtained by the medical use of medicinal plants is considerable. Therefore, the question that any physician trained in their use should ask is when will the public authorities introduce the courses in Clinical Phytotherapy into the curriculum of medical schools? More than ever, our country remains firmly opposed to any Phytotherapeutic research. And yet, our health system is creaking at the seams, economically and financially, but it also suffers from an ethical malaise.

The Servier scandal illustrates this moral crisis very well. Laboratoire Servier, the leading independent pharmaceutical company in France, and the second largest French pharmaceutical company worldwide, has been indicted for having concealed the true scale of the damaging effects of its medicinal products, and the number of deaths they have caused. The scandal revealed the scale of the conflict of interests that exist when experts on committees responsible for assessing drug safety are, at the same time, advisors and employees of the laboratories that they are supposed to be scrutinizing.

Knowing that drug companies cannot derive any financial benefit from the pharmaceutical use of medicinal plants is the most likely explanation for why they are being excluded from medical practice. As the effectiveness of medicinal plants comes to be recognized they will prove to be formidable competitors to synthetic molecules, and will represent a real challenge to the multinational drug companies.

But shouldn't the interests of the patient be paramount?

CHAPTER EIGHT

Debate surrounding the diseases of civilization

Two emblematic examples of the diseases of civilization: cholesterol and diabetes

The contemporary treatment and prevention of major diseases of civilization raises huge questions. We will limit our discussion to disorders of metabolism: excessive cholesterol and diabetes. As for cancer, this will be the subject of Chapter 10.

Cholesterol, can it really be public enemy number one?

For many years, cholesterol has been presented to the public and to the medical profession as an extremely dangerous substance for each of us. As one of the black sheep of healthcare, it is denounced as *the* indisputable risk to our arteries, and responsible for the scourge of cardiovascular disease, especially stroke and heart attacks, with all their disastrous consequences. Accordingly, it should be eliminated from our body at any price, and so it can be, thanks to the very potent medicinal products that have been developed and marketed by the pharmaceutical industry. But can such a negative view of cholesterol be justified considering that it is a substance that actually is indispensable to life?

Even if the correlation between abnormalities in the metabolism of cholesterol with an increased risk of fatal vascular accidents can be proven, these abnormalities are, however, only one of the risk factors among many others, which may be equally important.

The importance of lifestyle

Medicine has attributed the degradation of the walls of blood vessels to a wide range of interconnected causes, any of which might be implicated to a greater or lesser degree. So it is not only levels of triglycerides or cholesterol outside the normal range (a level of HDL lower than 0.35 g/L, and of LDL greater than 1.9 g/L) that may contribute to the deterioration of arteries. There are many other factors that play a considerable role: age and sex (from 45 years in men, 55 in women), family history of vascular disease, smoking (smoking over 20 cigarettes a day triples the coronary heart disease risk), hypertension, diabetes, excessive weight, abdominal obesity, and other nutritional factors. There are known behavioral contributors: excessive consumption of alcohol, a sedentary lifestyle with lack of regular physical activity, psychosocial stress, and other environmental factors. Other notable factors include disorders of coagulation, elevated level of certain inflammatory factors, hormonal treatments. It is worth pointing out that the heart rate itself is a strong predictor: the risk of sudden death is six times higher in a man whose heart rate is more than 88 per minute, as compared with one of less than 65.[1]

This data has been confirmed by the results of the international INTERHEART study,[2] which evaluated 30,000 patients from 52 countries from South and North America, Europe, Africa, Asia, and Australia. The study proves that in addition to the four known major factors of smoking, diabetes, hypertension, and hyperlipidemia, over 90% of myocardial infarctions are explained by five other factors that are also important: obesity, psychosocial stress, lack of sufficient daily intake of fruit and vegetables, lack of physical activity, and consumption of more than two glasses of wine per day. This data is important because it demonstrates that the overwhelming majority of heart attacks are attributable to these nine risk factors, and cannot be reduced solely to the level of cholesterol in the blood, as suggested by the simplistic equation: excess of cholesterol = heart in danger.

Cholesterol and triglycerides are essential to life

Before trying to get rid of substances considered dangerous, such as cholesterol and triglycerides, it might be a good idea to understand what role they play. Cholesterol belongs to the class of fatty compounds, or lipids, that constitute 15% of our body mass. The group includes free fatty acids, triglycerides, phospholipids, and steroids. Like any substance produced by the body, lipids have a specific purpose. They are the precursors of prostaglandins and leukotrienes, classes of compounds that play an important role in a wide range of bodily processes, from platelets and blood clotting to kidney function; they are also essential for inflammation and for the proper functioning of the immune system.

As cholesterol and triglycerides, like all fats, are poorly soluble in blood, the body uses carriers, known as lipoproteins. These are biochemical assemblies of proteins and lipids, which transport lipids to the tissues where they are needed. Some of these carriers, which transport cholesterol in the blood to cells that need it, may indeed be responsible for deposits in the walls of arteries. This is why they are said to be carriers of "bad" cholesterol (Low Density Lipoprotein or LDL-cholesterol). Others transport it to the liver, where it will be broken down into bile acids, and then excreted into the intestine: this is "good" cholesterol (HDL cholesterol).

Cholesterol is vital to life: we need it to construct the membranes of each and every cell in our body. Our cells can neither absorb nutrients nor eliminate waste unless these membranes, dependent on function properly. Because all the sex hormones (estrogen, progesterone, and testosterone) and the hormones of the adrenal gland (cortisol, aldosterone, and DHEA), are constructed from cholesterol, its importance cannot be overstated. It is crucial to the synthesis of other molecules, notably vitamin D, essential for bones, immunity, and cardiovascular health, as well as vitamin A. It creates the very structure and texture of the brain and participates in the branching and connectivity of neurons and synapse formation. It ensures the regeneration of nerve cells and the synthesis of neurotransmitters on which the propagation of the nerve impulse depends. In the brain, the neurons secrete just enough cholesterol to survive and develop, but not enough to establish connections between themselves. In order to manufacture these synapses, they need the cholesterol that is made by the neighboring glial cells. This phenomenon is vital, not only for the development of the brain, but also to repair connections destroyed by strokes or by neurodegenerative diseases such as Alzheimer's. Some researchers[3] think that a lack of cholesterol at the neuron level is probably involved in these kinds of disease.

By so forcibly reducing its level in the blood to such an extent, are we not in danger of artificially creating some new species of disease that may not be amenable to treatment? One may legitimately question the central and privileged place that modern medicine assigns to the drugs that help lower cholesterol, as if they were the only public health measure available for the prevention of cardiovascular disease.

A different approach: endobiogenic analysis of cholesterol and triglycerides abnormalities

Far from being a nuisance that should be eliminated at all costs, cholesterol plays a vital role in everyone. The Endobiogenic approach explains how the various properties of cholesterol (in common with other steroidal compounds) play a vital role in human metabolism, and is pivotal to all redox processes.[4] Accordingly, the body needs a well-orchestrated physiological strategy to process this crucial material from beginning to end. In the first place, absorption of nutrients from our diet must be regulated. Then, the subsequent synthesis of cholesterol in the liver as well as its eventual breakdown has to be managed in a precise way, as does its well-ordered elimination in the bile. Once we recognize the complexity of the mechanisms involved, we can understand how important a role the endocrine system plays[5] in the ordered management of cholesterol in the body.

Indeed, it has no choice other than be controlled by hormones, as it is these that regulate the metabolism of every substance in the body. Neither is it independent from the functional state of the organs that help build it (anabolize) or break it down (catabolize). These organs— intestines, liver, and pancreas—likewise have their functions managed by the endocrine system. Also, here as everywhere else in the human body, nothing can be dissociated and artificially isolated from the overall context of the patient. In the same way, the development and the fate of the cancerous cell at birth cannot be extricated from the whole being of the patient who may eventually suffer from cancer, cholesterol cannot be separated from the system to which it belongs: the body of the subject considered as a whole.

From this very different viewpoint, we can now make a more critical appraisal of those studies that demonize cholesterol as part of the war waged by the pharmaceutical industry in pursuit of selling their drugs.

Studies that we ought to look at again

The first study attempting to identify the factors that can contribute to the onset of cardiovascular diseases was conducted in 1948[6] in Framingham, a small town in the state of Massachusetts, on the eastern seaboard of the USA. It showed a statistical correlation between a high level of cholesterol in the blood and cardiovascular disease, but without fully taking account of other possible risk factors. Based on these findings, the level of total cholesterol not to be exceeded before andropause and menopause was set at 2.5 g/L, to which 0.10 g/L was then added for every 10 additional years of age. Over time, a great number of similar trials have been conducted with the consequence that the acceptable level of cholesterol has been gradually coming down, reaching 2.2 g/L in 1996, and then down to 2 g in 2006. This downward trend has, unsurprisingly, triggered an upward trend in the sale of the cholesterol-lowering products! Simple logic: as the normal level decreases, the number of people with higher than normal level will increase, as will the number of those needing medicinal products to get within those norms.

In July, 2002, the HPS study[7] even went so far as to conclude that, based on the results observed, simvastatin should be prescribed—*regardless of the cholesterol level in the blood*—to every individual suffering from coronary problems, or arteritis of the lower limbs, diabetes with at least one risk factor (a current or former smoker, for example), or anyone with a history of stroke. From now on, the prescription of simvastatin for these people will be automatic and inevitable. With this kind of thinking, one can envisage a situation where the demands of scientific research will in time require everybody to take synthetic medicinal products to eliminate any trace of cholesterol in our blood.

However, might such a move towards a kind of automated medicine, one that excludes the physician from any clinical decision or even from having to think at all, not become of itself a potential source of mistakes? If so, think of the great detriment to a huge number of people worldwide. Is it not the time to reconsider and reanalyze the results of numerous studies in the context of the individual and not based solely on statistical analysis, and to put the individual back at the heart of the goals of research?

A very profitable market

Given that the development of cardiovascular disease has truly a multitude of causes, it is curious that only cholesterol has been relentlessly pursued, when there are eight other factors that are equally implicated. Yet hardly a month goes by without the latest anti-cholesterol product making it into the headlines as yet another dramatic breakthrough. The economic motive behind pushing cholesterol into the public consciousness and to market is colossal. Atorvastatin,[8] for example, sold exclusively to reduce blood cholesterol, ranks first in the top ten best-selling medicinal products in the world.

This drug alone achieved a worldwide turnover of $10.7 billion in 2010 and has been acknowledged as the most profitable drug ever produced by the pharmaceutical industry. But the manufacturer Pfizer is currently faced with a serious problem: the patent, which protects its product in the United States, fell into the public domain in November, 2011. This means that less expensive generic drugs[9] can be quickly marketed by other laboratories, and thus threaten Pfizer's profits. According to the Wall Street Journal (August, 2011), the company seemed to have found a smart way out. All it has to do is re-brand atorvastatin as an "over-the-counter" (OTC) remedy, which means that it can be bought without a doctor's prescription. Selling it without prescription, treating it in the same way as aspirin, would help Pfizer boost its sales and resist the competition posed by generic medicines. For now, the position of the Food and Drug Administration (FDA), which alone can authorize such a re-categorization is unknown. Another example, Rosuvastatin,[10] developed by AstraZeneca and prescribed for hypercholesterolemia, was ranked tenth in 2010 with a turnover of $5.6 billion, up 26% on the previous year. The anti-cholesterol market is worth a veritable goldmine.

Some medical websites are solidly behind these drugs, and suggest that besides their cholesterol-lowering properties, they represent a new panacea for all manner of ills. One site reads: "more and more studies consistently show statins to have preventative effects against certain cancers; the risk of developing cancer of the lung, prostate, breast, pancreas, esophagus, or colon may be reduced by up to 50%."

Other sites suggest that as well lowering cholesterol, statins may also be effective against osteoporosis and may even protect the elderly from Alzheimer's. What are readers supposed to make of such an embarrassment of riches? Surely these claims must be genuine when they come from by a site developed by general practitioners and medical specialists? As these compounds are guaranteed to protect them against all these modern complaints, won't they be tempted to beg their doctor to prescribe them? Even a cursory glance at the length of the list of products marketed as combating high cholesterol might take you aback, and you would easily be overwhelmed when faced with the huge number of products in the Vidal Dictionary of French Medicaments, if you are currently healthy, but fear falling sick in the future. Let's take closer look.

These medicaments that modern science is selling to French customers, each having closely related biochemical structures, can effectively be divided into two major groups and more than 30 pharmaceutical companies are competing in the market.

The war against cholesterol waged by fibrate-based products

Fibrates[11] are medicinal products designed for patients for whom changes in lifestyle and diet have not adequately lowered their blood levels of triglycerides or cholesterol. They cause a significant reduction in the plasma concentration of triglycerides. Their precise mode of action at the molecular level has, until recently, been poorly understood. There are two major ways of lowering a substance in the blood, either by blocking its production, or increasing its rate of breakdown and elimination. This is how this type of medicine functions. It is currently known[12] that they act on the nuclear receptors capable of stimulating the transcription of genes that encoding the proteins involved in the metabolism of lipids and lipoproteins. Therefore, the use of these products exerts profound changes in the operation of complex systems, a fact that does not cross the mind of the clinician prescribing them and therefore no compensatory adjustment is made either. But these systems are necessarily connections with the workings of the whole body, and so the prescriber *should* be concerned about the consequences that such blocking may cause, both upstream and downstream of where they act.

No fewer than 19 laboratories promote these products.[13] Their usefulness was reassessed in October, 2010 by the European Medicines Agency, which concluded "the risk to benefit ratio of these medicines remains favorable, but they should be used only when treatment by statins is contraindicated or poorly tolerated." Vidal makes reference to the high frequency of side effects of these synthetic substances, such as: frequent digestive disorders and rash, headache, impotence, insomnia, dizziness; they tend to cause raised serum transaminase and gallstones, as well as muscle injuries, including the dreaded rhabdomyolysis.[14] Thus, it is legitimate to ask if their risk to ratio benefit really does lean toward the patient's benefit, and if treating one disorder only to create another one is in keeping with the Hippocratic maxim: "at least, do no harm." We are all the more entitled to question the validity of these treatments considering that their primary purpose, which is to reduce the mortality from cardiovascular disease, was put in considerable doubt by the findings of the Helsinki Heart Study.[15] This placebo-controlled, randomized study recruited 4,081 men between the ages of 40 and 55 with a high level of "bad" cholesterol, whether or not they also had an excess of triglycerides. When the number of deaths from all causes were analyzed, the medicinal product being trialed[16] did not demonstrate a positive outcome: 44 deaths in the treated group against 43 in the placebo group.

In addition, some of these medicinal products have been shown to increase the concentration of homocysteine in the blood. Now, homocysteine is an amino acid that is known to promote atherogenesis[17] and is precisely the process that the drug intervention was trying to prevent in the first place! The long-term adverse clinical consequences for cardiovascular disease of raised homocysteine levels can be serious. It is difficult to understand the rationale for prescribing a substance like fenofibrate[18] as a measure for reducing the risk of mortality from cardiovascular disease, when we know that it can raise the plasma concentration of homocysteine by as much as 50%.

Using statins to wage all-out war against cholesterol

Fundamental research for the development of new medicinal products continues unabated. The moment any new tiny biochemical mechanism comes under suspicion as possibly contributing to an excess of cholesterol, a new molecule is immediately sought to block it. Of course, finding a new way to attack cholesterol opens up a new niche in the market, and it is also good to get a lead on other companies because new patents are the way to dominate the market.

Ever on the lookout for some anomaly to block or to stimulate, researchers hit upon a choice physiological mechanism on which to act. They discovered that by inhibiting the action of the enzyme HMG-CoA reductase which controls the rate of synthesis of cholesterol in the liver, they were able to remove the "bad" cholesterol (LDL and VLDL) circulating in the arteries. They also observed a modest rise in "good" cholesterol (HDL), and so were able to kill two birds with one stone by removing the bad and elevating the good! They also found a direct correlation between dose and effect: the higher the dose of these statins, the more bad cholesterol was reduced, even up to a 50% reduction with high doses of the most potent compounds, such as atorvastatin. Raising the dose seems clinically justified in cases when a patient's cholesterol level refuses to drop.

A number of statins have come onto the market over time. They all act by blocking a specific function of the human body. Marketed in France by 26 companies, they can be split into five major groups. Lovastatin, the oldest (1987), heads the list of statins and is no longer marketed in France. Then simvastatin followed in 1988 (Lodales®, Simvastatin®, Zocor®), pravastatin in 1991 (Elisor®, Pravastatin®, Vasten®), Fluvastatin in 1994 (Fluvastatin®, Fractal®, Lescol®), atorvastatin in 1997 (Tahor®), and rosuvastatin in 2003 (Crestor®). Competition between laboratories is tough: no fewer than 20 of them are contending for the marketing of Pravastatin in France.

The gold-standard of modern medical is the placebo-controlled and double-blind clinical trials. These are conducted in many research centers all over the world and their findings are analyzed for their statistical effects. When a new product for lowering cholesterol in our arteries comes on to the market, its active molecule will be have been developed based on such trials. Medical science, conducted in this way, presents itself as the guarantor of the public health. Are these drugs, however, always good for our health?

Medicinal products that make people sick!

Having successfully completed the scientific requirements for any new drug as to safety and efficacy, Bayer Laboratories successfully obtained marketing authorization for cerivastatin,[19] but in 2001, after only four very profitable years on the market, this product was suddenly withdrawn from sale. Why was that?

In spite of the guarantees given by the Medicine Control Agencies, this particular statin proved to be responsible for very serious adverse effects, and caused more than a few deaths from rhabdomyolysis, a condition mentioned earlier. The true danger to life and health of these molecules, and the same goes for many other drugs on the market, don't always show up until they are used on a really massive scale. If only one adverse effect is reported for every 1,000 patients taking a certain medicinal product, the risk might at first seem quite low, but when 10 million people are taking the product, that means that 10,000 people will suffer the symptom. And when one of them is you, it means 100%! Also, given that each molecule can cause four or five other adverse effects, with a similar level of risk, duly listed by the laboratories, shouldn't we be alarmed at the number of people who will suffer from one or another of these side effects? It is alarming enough to read the list of potential side effects. All these secondary ills will in turn, of course, need to be treated by yet more drugs: an endless vicious circle leading to a proliferation of products.

Faced with these facts, we may well question the value of a medicine that claims to reduce the risk of developing one disease by prescribing products that sometimes cause others, some of them serious, in people who had nothing apparently wrong with them in the first place. And furthermore, some experts in the field consider that these prescriptions cannot be justified either in principle or in practice. Indeed, several researchers and physicians have seriously questioned the relevance and usefulness of statins. For example, in one of his books[20] in which he analyzes the problems raised by anti-cholesterol treatments, Dr. Michel de Lorgeril, cardiologist and researcher at the Department of Life Sciences of CNRS, calls into questions the role of cholesterol in cardiovascular disease. As a specialist in the prevention of these diseases, he argues that there is a lot of disinformation surrounding the real consequences to health of excess cholesterol. As a promoter of the Mediterranean diet, he accuses the pharmaceutical laboratories of deliberately misinterpreting the statistics concerning cardiovascular morbidity to justify the large-scale prescription of these very lucrative products. Coincidentally, fibrates or statins are reimbursed by the French social security system so if they are prescribed them, patients are also helped financially. After detailing the conflicts of interest between those experts in favor of statins and the pharmaceutical industry, Dr. de Lorgeril denounces what he calls "cholesterol delirium," by arguing that the war waged against cholesterol has failed to address the other risk factors, which we have already talked about, especially lifestyle and the Western diet, coupled with inadequate physical activity.

However, in France, taking a position that challenges powerful economic interests is not without risk. Dr. Marc Girard, European expert (AEXEA), who developed the first protocols in pharmacovigilance[21] and pharmaco-epidemiology,[22] has paid a price for adopting a critical stance towards the methods of evaluation that had been in use up till that time. Shortly after the Huriet Act on Biomedical Research (December, 1988), his name was included in the Register of Experts competent to testify in court in the field of Medicine and Biomedical Research. In this capacity, he testified in numerous public health cases, including a number of scandals that attracted huge media interest, such as: growth hormone, diethylstilbestrol, appetite suppressants, cerivastatin, the hepatitis B vaccine, glycol ethers, some of which he talked about in some of his books.[23] His name has since been removed from the Register of Experts following a campaign of harassment in the courts. His request for reinstatement on the Register has recently been turned down. It is not unreasonable to conclude that this refusal is a direct consequence of the position he has taken, particularly his demand that expert witnesses who are appointed to assess the benefits and risks of medicines should be truly independent from the pharmaceutical industry?

Bringing everyone in line with the standards

The objective of all cholesterol-lowering regimes is to bring the cholesterol of each individual into line with internationally agreed standards. Some have even floated the idea of adding cholesterol-lowering products to babies bottles to make sure they'll meet the standards later on in life. Is this not a tendency to reduce the complexity of life into a simplistic formula?

Surely, the circulating level of cholesterol, or glucose or whatever, can only be the outcome of an entire metabolic process. Consequently, to understand what a high or low level means, and what might have brought it about, we need to know and be able to analyze the various drives and constraints within the overall metabolism of any particular individual. In fact, an individual's cholesterol ensures not only the maintenance of function and structure, but it also the organism to respond to its adaptive needs, and so is not a true constant, in the strict sense of the term, and physiological variations is the true norm.

For this reason, setting a narrow universal band based on statistical predictions, which fails to take into account the specific structure of the individual nor the way this structure functions or adapts, and impose it on everybody, is to invite erroneous interpretations when it comes to the choice of the appropriate treatment. For example, in cases where a cholesterol level above the statistical norm reflects an adaptive response to a metabolic demand in a subject should not be forcibly lowered, as an inopportune treatment would only aggravate the individual's condition. As physicians, we are all familiar with elderly patients who have had a high cholesterol level for over 30 or 40 years, but whose arteries are in perfect condition, as we are with young people with low cholesterol, who, by contrast, have damaged and sclerotic arteries. This just goes to show that each individual has their own unique metabolism and that the key to the prevention of cardiovascular disease may not lie with strict standardization, and even less with the blanket prescription of cholesterol-lowering substances for everybody. This is particularly true in subjects over 75 years of age who may already be taking a number of medicines, and for whom it is recognized that the risk of not having enough cholesterol is greater than having it in excess.

On the subject of risk, some international scientific publications are beginning to connect the use of statins to force down levels of so-called "bad" cholesterol (LDL) with an increased risk of developing certain types of cancer.[24] Other studies have reported an increase in the risk of attempted suicide.[25]

The endobiogenic approach to the patient with high cholesterol level: identifying the true causes

An Endobiogenic physician does not make blanket prescriptions but rather adapts the treatment to each patient as an individual after carefully evaluating his or her particular metabolic state, which may be entirely different to that of another patient who is similar only in having a high level of cholesterol.

When examining an individual presenting with an abnormally high level of bad cholesterol or triglycerides, or too low a level of good cholesterol, the doctor should first reflect and examine the patient from every angle and try to understand what this abnormality means in this particular case. Nothing in the body occurs by chance, so the doctor has to find the "hidden variables" behind the blood test results by assessing the state of the liver and the intestines, as well as, most importantly, the functioning of the endocrine system. This, after all, manages energy needs and the anabolism and catabolism of all the substances necessary for life, as well as maintaining triglycerides as a reserve source of energy.

Only when these factors have been correctly identified and understood, can an appropriate treatment plan be formulated and one that will be tailored to the individual rather than to the apparently abnormal blood test.

Resist prescribing blindly

There are, of course, times when a symptomatic treatment is justified, but only in cases where the body is genetically incapable of metabolizing cholesterol normally, because of an abnormality, for example, in the gene that codes for the LDL receptor.[26] Symptomatic treatment with a synthetic molecule may also be considered from time to time in patients who are inherently at high risk and whose level of dysfunction is also high. Even with these cases, a careful assessment of the risk to benefit ratio of the prescribed drug should be undertaken, and a treatment adapted to the terrain should be prescribed concurrently. But in no case should a doctor make a prescription on the basis of statistical evidence alone, with all the paradoxes entailed.

Blocking cholesterol production will lead to an accumulation of other compounds upstream of this blockade, with unknown consequences. To interfere artificially with a biological system that is already in some kind of parlous state, without even having looked into the true cause of the anomalous cholesterol, can hardly be the right clinical solution.

A few questions to ask

In any given case, does the raised cholesterol reflect the body's response to an excessive demand for production of genital hormones, for example? If so, the cholesterol excess can only be resolved after the explanation for this high demand has been understood. Is the excess caused by eating too many fatty foods? If so, the diet needs to be addressed. Or is the excess caused from the body's inability to burn fat? If so, the hormonal reasons for this inability should be sought, and appropriately treated. Or are the systems of elimination or the excretory organs impaired or overloaded so that their capacity to process wastes is overwhelmed? If that is the case, the treatment will be quite different from the previous situations.

If you really want to provide the patient with a solution that is tailored to their particular circumstances, there are many other similar questions that need to be asked. The answers inevitably lead to personalized therapeutic decisions, specific to each individual. The patient can be told: "yes, your cholesterol is high *but* this is the consequence of an entire set of imbalances which are specific to you, and *therefore* it is not so much your cholesterol that needs be dealt with, but rather the correction of the imbalances that caused them." This is in marked contrast to the current approach that generalizes every case to the same: "yes, your cholesterol is high, and *therefore* you must immediately take this medicine to bring it down."

Dietary solutions proposed for lowering cholesterol

The major dietary contributors to the reduction of cardiovascular disease risk are now well known. In line with the Mediterranean diet, they settle, to an extent, the question of foods that may be deleterious to the human body and so provides an opportunity for the number of dietary stressors to be reduced. By reducing the intake of saturated fats of animal origin (butter and dairy products, meat, deli meats, and eggs), and favoring foods rich in unsaturated fats such as olive or rapeseed oils, fatty fish such as herring, mackerel, and sardines, poultry and fruits, nuts and seeds almonds, hazelnuts, walnuts, olives, and avocado, and vegetables, rich in antioxidants, we can reduce the levels of cholesterol and triglycerides in the blood.

Nonetheless, in spite a reduction in the intake of dietary fats to 35% of the caloric intake and of dietary cholesterol to less than 300 mg/day, and a qualitative change in the fatty acid intake by reducing saturated fatty acids in favor of monounsaturated and polyunsaturated fatty acids, cholesterol levels are often reduced by only a very small amount. Many people, even after following an onerous diet, are not rewarded for all their effort, and their cholesterol level remains stubbornly high.

There is no mystery about this once one understands that it is the body itself that manages its own level of cholesterol. A person with abnormalities in the metabolism and elimination of cholesterol will persist in producing an excess even if starved almost to death unless a therapeutic strategy is implemented that aims to correct the underlying imbalance.

A new approach to diseases related to cholesterol abnormalities

We know that damaged arteries are the greatest predictors of cardio-vascular accidents because damaged arteries lose their flexibility and elasticity, their tone and their integrity. When circulating blood contains inflammatory substances, a lesion can gradually build up at the site of a damaged arterial wall. Over time, the lesion deteriorates, and the artery becomes sclerotic. The stage is set for calamitous events such as strokes and infarcts to occur, which are the inevitable consequence of a tissue chronically deprived of oxygen. Cardiovascular or cerebrovascular accidents are poorly named: far from happening by accident, they are the inevitable result of the poor state of the artery and of the blood and the resultant malfunction and dysregulation.

The doctor, therefore, has to bear in mind all the diverse elements that influence the state of the artery wall and contribute to the formation of an atheromatous plaque and to formulate a treatment capable of acting on the arterial lining as well on the abnormalities in the circulating blood. These factors include the state of the endothelial cells and vascular reactivity, muscle cell proliferation, and the presence of extracellular matrix and degrading enzymes called metalloproteases. Inflammatory compounds and factors of immunity in the blood must be considered as well as abnormalities in its lipid profile. To understand them fully, we should try to uncover any imbalances in the functioning of the autonomic nervous system. We should do the same for the entire endocrine system, with emphasis on the thyroid and reproductive hormones, as well as insulin, growth hormone, and the hormones of the adrenal glands: these will all be implicated in the degradation of the arterial wall. Of course, we must also evaluate the functioning of the organs of detoxification and elimination, such as the liver, intestines, and kidneys.

We must strive, therefore, to cover both problems at the same time by treating the arterial wall and balancing the composition of the blood. This is only possible if the doctor takes into account not only the state of the arteries and the blood but also places these organs within the context of all the systems that manage them. If we try to only lower cho-lesterol, we are very far from resolving the real source of the problems.

This is the comprehensive strategy offered by Endobiogeny towards cardiovascular disease and to those who have to live with its effects.

Examples of treatment

To illustrate the difference between a symptomatic and an integrative approach based on modern science, here is the case of a patient with a high level of cholesterol, suffering from the effects of arteriosclerosis.

This 60-year-old man is 1.68 meters tall and weighs 85 kilos, and so is considered obese. He eats out in restaurants every day and feels overwhelmed by his professional responsibilities. He does not take any regular exercise. He comes for a consultation because he is concerned about the results of a blood test which show his fasting blood glucose to be 1.26 g/L, his total cholesterol 2.85 g, with a cholesterol/HDL ratio of 5.8; his LDL is 1.95 and triglycerides are 2.20 g/L; his blood pressure is 140/90. He is even more concerned because, while his electrocardiogram at rest is normal, his cardiac stress test is not good. His myocardial scintigraphy came back normal, but the fact that his father died of a myocardial infarction at age 66 preys on his mind.

Conventional treatment

His own doctor suggested he follow a standard dietary regime and, following current guidelines, prescribed the following treatment, with the following aims:

– Metformin®, 1 tablet in the morning and 1 in the evening (to lower blood glucose)
– Zocor® 20 mg, 1 tablet in the evening (to lower blood cholesterol)
– Atenolol® 100 mg, 1 tablet in the morning (a beta blocker to lower blood pressure)
– Chlorothiazide® 500, 1 tablet in the morning (a diuretic to lower blood pressure).

Endobiogenic treatment

The treatment plan was based on a comprehensive approach of the patient's case.[27] Following a clinical examination, it was decided that the prescription should include whole-plant extracts in order to be able to fully meet the following objectives:

- to slow down the activity of the alpha-sympathetic and beta-sympathetic branches of the nervous system
- to ensure better renal flow in order to lower the blood pressure
- to decrease the level of endogenous stress
- to promote relaxation of the arterial tone by a direct action on smooth muscle
- to regulate blood glucose by improving pancreatic function, both exocrine and endocrine
- to diminish the activity of growth hormone, as this may be a risk factor for arteriosclerosis
- to provide a rich source of silica, with its proven action in preventing arterial degeneration (by using horsetail powder, for example)
- to support detoxification and drainage by the liver and to increase the lipid-lowering functions of the body and so mitigate the negative effects of obesity
- to reduce the negative effects of excessive oxidation on the arterial system
- to reduce the tendency for blood clotting and so reduce the risk of thrombosis in this man, whose father died of a heart attack.

The treatment outlined below is based on fundamental research (with which the prescribing physician needs to be well acquainted) that demonstrates that, among its other actions, essential oil of lavender (*Lavandula officinalis*) possesses:

- hypotensive properties, by virtue of its activity on both the alpha-sympathetic and beta-sympathetic branches of the nervous system
- anticoagulant properties
- increases the production and flow of bile in the liver and into the intestine

Additionally, horsetail (*Equisetum arvense*) has anti-sclerotic properties largely on account of its organic silica content.

The prescription

The patient was given two liquid preparations and five dry medicinal products as listed below. All were to be taken twice daily, morning and evening, ten minutes before breakfast and dinner.

- 70 drops of Preparation A mixed with 100 drops of Preparation B in a little water,
- 2 tablets prepared from dry extracts of birch, olive tree, and fumitory,
- 1 capsule prepared from walnut and plantain,
- 1 capsule of evening primrose oil,
- 1 teaspoon of powder of horsetail,
- 1 vial of granions of selenium.

PREPARATION A
- essential oil of lavender (*Lavandula officinalis*) 4 g
- essential oil of clary sage (*Salvia sclarea*) 2 g
- *Tilia tomentosa* buds as glycerin macerate D1 enough to bring the total to 125 ml.

PREPARATION B
- equal quantities of the following, bringing the total to 125 ml
- fluid extract of *Cimicifuga racemosa*
- fluid extract of *Poterium sanguisorba*
- fluid extract of *Medicago sativa*

Two months later, the patient's cholesterol level had dropped from 2.85 to below 2.30, with normal triglycerides; his blood glucose is within normal range; his blood pressure at rest is 130/80. The patient feels himself to be in very good shape and has not experienced any unwanted effects. He has recovered his *joie de vivre*. All things considered, does this amount to a "cure," and how should we manage his follow-up?

As with any symptom, whether biological (excess of cholesterol) or functional (migraines, for example), just because the symptom has disappeared we cannot assume that the patient is cured! The physician must always support his or her assessment, not only on the patient's subjective report, but backed up by a careful physiological follow-up, integrating close clinical study with biological evaluation.[28]

For every patient and for each examination, the doctor should constantly question both the diagnosis and the treatment, whether based on synthetic chemical, medicinal plants, diet, or any other modality. Above all, the needs of the patient must be first and foremost, which is far from easy, considering the complexity of the human being. This flies in the face of the current trend of prescribing standardized treatments— said to be best practice—given that everyone now recognizes the real and significant toxicity that may attend them. This often means that patients run risks at least as serious as those from which we would hope to protect them. It seems reasonable that doctors should prescribe the least toxic treatments and reserve highly potent synthetic molecules for those who really need them.

Proposals for the future

The stakes are high in current medical practice; the example of cholesterol may be extended to all other areas of disease. Many independent experts warn that the influence of the pharmaceutical industry on this huge field of disorders of lipid and cholesterol metabolism is such that it blocks any political will to call for large-scale clinical trials to discover the medicinal products with the best cost to benefit ratio and the lowest toxicity.

The use of lipid-lowering medication as preventative in patients with high cholesterol but who do not suffer from cholesterol-related disease seems to be the accepted norm, in spite of all the reported side effects. Given how powerful they are, their place as preventatives in patients with normal cholesterol and who suffer no side effects is much more troubling, especially in those with low or moderate risk. The absence of a marked reduction on overall mortality leads us to propose the use of medicinal plants as first line therapeutic agents for these millions of patients whose condition does not justify the use of aggressive therapy. Based on the results obtained by the many doctors using them successfully in their daily practice, we ask that real studies be conducted in our hospitals to assess the benefits to the people in their care.

Another major public health problem: diabetes

Diabetes, a costly sugar

Type-2 diabetes, or so-called maturity onset diabetes, is mostly found in overweight or obese subjects. It is one of the most widespread diseases of civilization and could potentially affect 370 million people over the next 20 years. It is the result of an impaired insulin response, which is no longer able to regulate the level of glucose in the blood effectively. When the level of this hormone is inadequate or if it no longer functions normally, the blood glucose rises inexorably. A state of continual excess of glucose in the blood damages the arteries and capillaries, and may lead to long-term complications in the micro-vasculature. The tissues most vulnerable to damage are the tiny blood vessels in the retinas, kidneys and nerve cells, and also those in the heart and brain so the disease predisposes to heart attack, arteritis and stroke, responsible for a rising number of deaths.

Widely regarded as one of the consequences of our modern unbalanced and stressful lifestyle and dietary habits that tend to obesity, this disease places a huge burden on healthcare budgets throughout the world. In France, the number of patients treated for diabetes was estimated to have been nearly 4% of the population in 2007, or over 2,500,000 people.[29] Reimbursements from healthcare insurance to people with diabetes were evaluated at €12.5 billion, or approximately 8% of the total reimbursement expenditure. The increase in the average annual cost of a treatment per diabetic patient, for all types of care, increased by 30% between 2001 and 2007. Given the magnitude of these costs, and the increase in the number of the treatments prescribed during this period, it would seem like a good idea to take stock of how well the new treatments have performed over these years.

The classical approach of the fatal complications of diabetes and the Avandia scandal

It is unusual these days to die of a diabetic coma and this is one of the great achievements of modern medicine. Advances in resuscitation techniques have helped save diabetic patients from certain death at a critical phase in their disease, or in case of acute hyperglycemia. Chronic disease, however, is the cause of numerous serious complications and so constitutes a real crisis in public health.

In trying to reduce deaths and morbidity from type-2 diabetes, modern medicine considers that its primary task should be to lower levels of blood glucose, so you will be classed as diabetic if your fasting blood glucose level exceeds the maximum level set at 1.26 g/L. The reason for this threshold is that this is level at which destruction of micro-vessels starts to occur, increasing the risk of complications. Diabetic disease is, therefore, defined by the complications it generates, and not, as we should be entitled to expect, by an explanation of the mechanisms by which the body lost its ability to manage the uptake of glucose into the cells. This means that we ignore from the outset the real causes of the disease, located upstream of the glucose circulating in the blood. The classic approach will be hell-bent on the elimination of the aggressor: the excessive glucose level, held responsible for the fatal complications. If that is truly so, then it would seem reasonable to assume that the more we lower the glucose level, the greater the chances to avoid such complications.

This is the focus of current medical research. To accomplish this goal, it was decided to prescribe more potent treatments to bring down the blood glucose within statistically determined levels. The very first sign of a symptom is pounced upon and a treatment program put in place with every effort is made to bring it down as low as possible in the hope of averting diabetic lesions. Stronger and stronger medicinal products are prescribed in the hope of bringing down the number of deaths! Numerous studies, based on the most up-to-date science, have been conducted to critically and quantitatively evaluate the correctness of this approach.

Thus, ACCORD (Action to Control Cardiovascular Risk in Diabetes Study Group) studied 10,251 diabetic patients. After 3.5 years of follow-up, it has not only proven that the rate of serious hypoglycemia and weight gain (of over 10 kilos) were significantly higher in the group undergoing intensive therapy, but more importantly, that the mortality was higher in this group than in the patients treated with lower doses of medicinal products. Because of this, the study had to be prematurely stopped. Another study, VADT (Veteran Affairs Diabetes Trial), which studied 1,791 patients in 20 North American centers devoted to army veterans, came to the same conclusions. After 6 years of follow-up, even though the more reliable marker that tracks the longer-term glucose trend (known as HbA1c) had successfully improved, the rate of major cardiovascular events in the two groups of patients turned out to have been identical. The study additionally confirmed the very high incidence of severe hypoglycemia reported in the ACCORD study, with a higher number of sudden deaths in the group undergoing intensive therapy. Such data warranted further larger scale research, as other studies seemed to report conflicting findings. Dr. Catherine Cornu (Center of Clinical Investigations, Inserm-Lyon) and her collaborators conducted a meta-analysis published in 2011.[30] This method is considered very reliable; it involves collating results and analyzing data from all comparable studies using sophisticated statistical tools. The work focused on 34,533 patients, of whom 18,315 had undergone intensive

therapy while 16,218 had received the standard treatment. The aim of
the meta-analysis was to discover whether the greater drop in blood
glucose brought about by intensive anti-diabetic treatments correlated
with a reduction in the overall number of cardiovascular accidents.
Given the rationale behind the intensive approach, one might reasonably have expected a positive correlation, but that was not to be the case.

The failure of the anticipated results to show up demonstrates yet
again the shortcomings of the reductionist view. By limiting itself to
the elimination of a single biological finding, excessive blood glucose in
this case, and failing to take into account the particularity in the overall state of the individual, it has to face the facts of biological reality.
The meta-analysis of 13 studies showed that intensive therapy of type-2
diabetes, has little effect, when compared with the standard treatment,
on mortality from all causes, including those of cardiovascular origin.
This means that it can serve no purpose to increase the dose of medication as doing so fails to reduce the death-rate attributable to diabetes.[31]
In short, the study attests to the failure of an aggressive therapy that
has been imposed equally on all sufferers. Furthermore, some modest progress in a non-life-threatening condition comes at the price of
a considerable increase in the risk of inducing another disease, which
in some cases may prove fatal. Not to mention the multiple secondary
effects, which may not yet be fully known, and may show up many
years from now, in various guises, depending on the individual. If one
had hoped for promising outcomes for people with the disease, they
were not forthcoming.

We should not fail to mention the case of rosiglitazone. Licensed as
safe as an anti-diabetic compound, it was marketed in 2000 as Avandia
by GSK Laboratory in Europe, where it enjoyed a great deal of publicity.
Heralded as a preventative against the complications posed by diabetic
micro-angiopathy, it therefore gained an important place in the doctors'
arsenal of modern medicines. It was not long before its negative effects
became obvious, and doctors who had prescribed it promptly made
their findings known. But, curiously, it took almost 10 years before
AFSSAPS and the European Medicines Agency banned the drug. The
Agency eventually recognized that, contrary to the claims made by its
manufacturers, this drug is associated with a higher risk of myocardial
infarction and strokes than other anti-diabetic treatments. The remedy
actually induced diseases that it was supposed to cure! Rosiglitazone
reported sales of $2.2 billion in 2006. In 2009, after its serious side effects

had already been published, the reported sales were "only" $1.2 billion. In 2010/2011, almost 110,000 people were still taking it daily.

How much confidence can we have in the conclusions drawn from studies conducted by professors of international renown, the authorities in their field?[32] In July, 2010, B. Zinman and his collaborators published some remarkable results in the *Lancet*[33] that found that the combination therapy of rosiglitazone (Avandia) and metformin was remarkably effective in preventing the development of type-2 diabetes in subjects with glucose intolerance, and with very few side effects. Yet this same rosiglitazone had been placed under surveillance in July, 2010, and withdrawn from the market in November, 2010,[34] for having caused serious vascular problems. Whom should we believe? How many more Avandias, praised today will tomorrow be withdrawn for safety reasons?

Findings like this challenge our current approach to the prevention of the deadly complications of diabetes, and led *Le Quotidien du médecin* of July 27, 2011, to run an editorial entitled: "Paradoxes of Intensive Therapy for Type 2 Diabetes." Indeed, it would be difficult not to find such results paradoxical. But above all, how can they be explained by current physiological knowledge? Is there some alternative we can recommend to our patients?

The endobiogenic approach to diabetes

Diabetes is a disease in which insulin is unable to maintain the blood glucose within normal range and is therefore considered to be a disease of the insulin-secreting cells of the pancreas. In type-1 diabetes (in which these cells have been destroyed), the aim of treatment is simply to remedy the situation by administering insulin by injection. In type-2 diabetes, which is the focus of our discussion here, there is a generalized metabolic failure of the action of the hormone insulin on the body as a whole.

As type-2 diabetes is a condition very commonly associated with other serious problems such as hypertension and abnormal blood lipids, which will in turn exacerbate the vascular complications of the diabetes, conventional treatment tends to manage each of these symptoms as they arise, without any comprehensive attempt to analyze the physiological relations between the various functions and the disturbances giving rise to all the signs. To focus exclusively on insulin and ignore the overall hormonal context of the individual is to oversimplify the true state of affairs. To take a wider approach to the issue, it is first necessary to consider the role glucose plays in the body and what systems are in place to manage it.

Glucose is the main energy source for all the cells in the body. The human brain is the organ that consumes the largest share: 120 g/day for an adult person and 80 g/day for a 1-year-old child. Glucose could be likened to the fuel injected into an engine, enabling the body to run all the metabolic processes, whether they are catabolic, breaking down, and making material available, or anabolic, using these materials to build and maintain necessary structures. Just as a car needs gasoline to run the engine, so the oxidation of glucose provides the energy needed for chemical reactions. But glucose and insulin are by no means the only agents involved: we saw in Chapter 3 that insulin is a hormone that belongs to the somatotropic axis, which is, ultimately, the axis in charge of the construction of tissues. However, I am sure that by now you will have understood that this one axis is not independent of the other axes that make up the endocrine system, which constitutes the true manager of the whole body.

So we must consider the complex activities of these axes to understand their contribution to the regulation of glucose. By taking into account the influence of cortisol, estrogens, thyroid, and growth hormones, as well as the autonomic nervous system, we will obviously broaden our understanding of the disease and the way we manage it. We must also consider the digestive organs that regulate glucose: the intestines where it is absorbed from food, the liver where it is stored. All of these play their part in helping insulin maintain the level of glucose within normal range. Faced with two patients with a high glucose level, the doctor has to identify the source of their insulin failure in order to treat each of them effectively.

Whether the doctor treating diabetes takes a conventional or an Endobiogenic approach, both are faced with the same reality: that the disease is always a question of insulin. However, one focuses only on the pathology while the other contextualizes it within the totality of the patient. Accordingly, the therapeutic choices made by the latter will be very different in principle and applied in an integrative manner. This broader approach will help us understand why some diabetic patients will develop early vascular complications, while others will not develop them for many years. Given all this, and the serious challenge posed by diabetes, medicinal plants provide a helpful resource towards the prevention, treatment and management of this disease, for the benefit of patients and society at large.

Example of patient treatment

The conventional approach to diabetes

This widespread disease is dangerous on account of the cardiovascular damage caused by the chronically high levels of glucose in the blood; if untreated, it may also cause kidney disease and retinal damage. The cause is considered to be the consequence of an abnormal regulation of glucose by insulin.

The aim of conventional treatment is to bring down the high level of glucose in the blood and maintain it within the normal range. A one-size fits all approach offers an anti-symptom medicine to quell the one symptom. In this case, an excess glucose is treated by an anti-glucose medicinal product, or by adding insulin.

Diabetes: endobiogenic approach

That there is an excess of glucose in the blood is not in doubt. Of course, this excess is harmful to the patient, but the problems are not limited to the damage that excess glucose can cause. other systems and factors are implicated and these may amplify the risks of damage, especially to small blood vessels. The Endobiogenic approach requires the physician to view the diabetic patient in a radically different way. The first thing to say is that glucose is connected with numerous functions and is situated between the activity of other organs, such as the liver and intestines. These participate in its regulation, and therefore the functional state of these organs must be taken into consideration.

Treatment therefore should take into account the overall physiological state of the individual. An excess of glucose in the blood is only but one indicator of an imbalance caused by certain abnormalities that are peculiar to each individual diabetic patient. The physician should therefore consider the state of the intestines that transport glucose into different parts of the body, as well as the liver that stores and releases it, (under the influence of glucagon secreted by the pancreas). Glucocorticoid hormones from the adrenal cortex will influence the interconversions between sugars, fats and proteins; levels of adrenaline will greatly influence the need for the mobilization of blood sugar. The other element to be addressed is how well the tissues with a high need for glucose are functioning, and how well it is processed inside those cells under the control of various hormones.

All of this requires us to make a comprehensive assessment of the production and consumption of glucose as well as the management of insulin by the body, as it is the only hormone able to take glucose from the blood and transfer it into the cell, all others having effectively the opposite effect. In addition to the concepts of interrelation and function, Endobiogeny also addresses the dynamics. It considers that life is not static and since adaptation is a permanent phenomenon, the level of elements circulating in our blood (sugar, in this example) varies according to demand; this aspect must be taken into consideration before responding to any blood test results. The conventional approach has set strict levels for glucose, as it has for cholesterol and other substances, and these norms are the same for everyone; they take no account of the fact that the human body is not static, but in permanent movement. In doing so, it ignores the fact that each body has its own needs and sets its own standards, and wanting to force it into a statistical standard, may sometimes open the door to negative consequences. Such an approach denies the reality of the constant adaptation that takes place within our bodies. A blood glucose level that is a little higher than normal may simply indicate a response to a greater energy need, more or less transient, that can only be met by an increased level of sugar. If this excess is due to an adaptation attempt mounted by the body in response to a need, forcing it down artificially is likely to frustrate this process and lead to a negative outcome. A more cogent treatment would involve understanding this need and addressing it accordingly. It would appreciate that the cause of a disease does not necessarily originate where it is expressed, and so the site where it is expressed should not necessarily be the place to treat it.

To conclude this chapter devoted to two major diseases of civilization, we will touch upon another big problem that affects us all: the threat of the endocrine disruptors.

Endocrine disruptors and our health

"Endocrine Disruptors in the Spotlight" read the headline of an article in *Le Figaro* in July, 2011. The risks posed to our health by chemical substances released into the environment have become better known and are a legitimate source of concern. Each of us is constantly exposed to thousands of synthetic products, each of which can potentially interact with our own endocrine system, posing a real health problem. As we have already mentioned on several occasions, the endocrine system manages and controls the metabolic state of our body. It is in charge of the growth and development of organs and our immune system, our reproduction and how we mobilize energy, and maintain homeostasis. It is the omnipresent guardian of our body and the guarantor of our health.

Unfortunately, the majority of chemical substances present in our environment behave as endocrine disruptors, which is to say that by they act on our hormonal system to disrupt its normal functioning.[35] They adversely affect the mechanisms which regulate cell division and growth. They are also able to inhibit the aspects of the immune system, by blocking the activity of T lymphocytes, and by reducing the number of NK cells (natural killer cells), which are essential elements of our defense against infection. By modifying the major control mechanisms of the body, these endocrine disruptors have the capability of inducing abnormalities with incalculable consequences for the health and the fate of the human race. They may cause a whole range of diseases: some cancers, degenerative diseases, allergies, disordered immunity, genital malformations, and loss of fertility. In addition, altering the normal sequences of the endocrine axes (see Chapter 3), they will almost certainly give rise to "orphan diseases" which have yet to be assigned their true cause. And these phenomena are even more serious when these molecules are absorbed during pregnancy, or by infants and young children in the early stages of development.

These compounds are disruptive at very low doses, and they may have other, as yet unknown and cumulative effects, which may show up many years hence. Thus, it is important to take into account the duration of exposure, because the true extent of their toxicity may take decades to make itself known, and may even skip one or more generations before showing up in our descendants.

Does current legislation protect us?

These endocrine disruptors are concealed in a wide range of products found in everyday life, in our food, and even in medicines.[36] Modern science knows very little about their additive effects when several of them are absorbed at the same time, especially during phases of growth and hormonal transition. This potential synergy makes them even more dangerous. Unknowingly, we are continually absorbing a whole range of toxic compounds, which are accumulating in our bodies and in our tissues. We breathe them, swallow them, or apply them to our skin. Coming from agricultural, urban, or domestic pollution, our food, medicines, and cosmetic products are all contaminated.

It should therefore come as no surprise that the commission of experts appointed to examine the regulation of such disruptors, would make the recommendation that "products containing compounds with a clear risk of endocrine disruption should be subject to special labeling, warning mothers and encouraging them to use another product."[37]

If these substances are indeed dangerous, should we be satisfied with such paltry measures? Rather than simply labeling a product as dangerous, why not simply withdraw it from sale? Tackling this issue of the regulation of industrial products, most of which are dangerous for human health because of these endocrine disruptors, is a perilous undertaking: powerful vested interests are in conflict with consumer groups. On the one hand, we have the chemical industry, which will do everything it can to pressurize the regulatory authorities into keeping its compounds on the market. On the other, consumer groups with legitimate concerns about the risks such products pose to human health. Looking at the better-known cases that have come to light, you come to realize that financial and economic interests always take precedence over consumers' health, and that only scandals such as that involving Mediator®, can shift things a little. It may take decades for a product to be withdrawn from the market from the time that researchers flag up harmful effects.

It is difficult to resist making a connection between the regulatory bodies charged with the surveillance of environmental products and those, such as AFSSAPS, which up until 2011 regulated medicinal products.[38] There are so many ways and means that industrial power can frustrate and delay regulatory decisions, including covert pressures on the authorities and because of concealed conflicts of interest: some of those in charge of marketing decisions are in the pay of chemical industries or of pharmaceutical companies.

As soon as a study flags up a potential risk posed by a compound, the "experts" try to discredit the research by maintaining that it had not been properly conducted, that the statistical analysis of the data was inconclusive and could be open to a different interpretation. It all takes time, deadlines get pushed back, and all the evidence and counter arguments get lost in the labyrinthine corridors of bureaucracy. The outcome is biased towards invalidating the study or tempering its interpretation of risk. In the end, the decision to allow the incriminated product to remain on sale is "justified" because it is deemed to pose "a low risk, on account of the weak concentration of toxic compounds." They refuse to concede that long-term hazards might exist, and even if there did, they could be attributed to causes other than the suspected product. Animal studies are dismissed, as inapplicable to humans because "even if there is evidence of risk in animals, there is no convincing evidence in humans." For those who are more concerned with the health of their contemporaries than the prosperity of multinationals in the chemicals sector, the task is made all the more difficult because they do not hold the keys to power of decision-making.

CHAPTER NINE

Carol's case: metastatic breast cancer

The story of carol, an american patient, suffering from breast cancer

On Christmas Eve in 1997, Carol Silverander, a lively blonde in her 50s, learned that she had breast cancer. It came as a shock for this vegetarian, healthy, and active woman. However, doctors at the Cedar-Sinai Hospital in Los Angeles were at pains to reassure her that this "would soon be over." Her oncologist predicted that this would be speedily cleared up by surgery and radiotherapy, leaving nothing but a bad memory. Carol was full of hope and happy to take in these soothing words. Unfortunately, less than 2 years later, she discovers that her "insignificant cancer, brief incident" had spread to the liver and the bones.

Her oncologists now gave her chance of survival beyond 2 years as less than 5%, based on US official statistics. Carol's story is not at all unusual, and many women have lived through similar experiences.

Her primary cancer was thought to be quite a "small" tumor

In 1996, she was 51 years old and still having regular periods. She was in good health and there was nothing at all to trouble her. Her gynecologist gave her the standard advice ahead of her menopause, which was to take hormone replacement therapy (HRT), in the form of an estrogen and progesterone pill.

Such prescriptions are usually justified along the following lines: "We can now substitute those hormones which will be diminished when your periods stop so that you won't have to put up with all the unpleasant symptoms. We can prevent drying of the skin and mucous membranes, and we will help you keep your figure longer. You won't be waking up at night drenched in sweat nor have hot flashes by day. You can look forward to a good stable mood, because our modern medicines will help you avoid the depression to which all postmenopausal women are prone. In addition, they protect your bones, which become more fragile with the drop of estrogen over time, and so your risk of femoral neck fracture, for example, is reduced. The doses are very safe now and the risks minimal, going by the statistics. The benefits will be far greater than all the problems that you will certainly encounter if you do not take the hormones."

Given these assurances, Carol doesn't hesitate to embark on the course of treatment, and why not? She doesn't want to deprive herself of the opportunities offered by modern medicine to stay young as long as possible and doesn't want to lose her dynamic personality, which helps her handle her weighty professional responsibilities.

Unfortunately, 18 months later, in December, 1997, while washing, she discovers a lump in her left breast. While cysts are commonly found in the breast of a young women, given the hormonal changes of their menstrual cycle, the same finding in a peri-menopausal woman, and under hormonal treatment, is an important warning sign that needs to be urgently investigated.

Very quickly, everything goes into overdrive. Her gynecologist is very concerned and orders a whole battery of standard tests: mammogram, ultrasound, CT scan, MRI scan, scintigraphy, blood tests, cancer markers, and finally a biopsy, which confirms the diagnosis:

"The results are not good. You have cancer, but fortunately your tumor is very small and was found early. I will send you to be seen by my specialist team. The surgeon is excellent and I think you will be left with only a small scar. Then, depending on the results of the microscopic analysis of the tumor, the oncologists will decide the follow-up treatment. Thanks to the progress we have made in treating cancer, this kind of tumor is easily treated these days. A short ordeal, and you will come back to see me in a month in top form."

These reassuring words would prove to be entirely inadequate in dealing with this very real disease.

Surgery in such cases usually involves removing the tumor and a large part of the surrounding tissue, up to half the breast. It is normal also to remove the lymph nodes in the armpit in case the cancer has spread, which is associated with a less good prognosis. In Carol's case, nine lymph nodes were removed and, fortunately, they all turned out to be negative. In March, 1998, she had radiotherapy to her thorax and her left armpit, with the aim of destroying any cancer cells that might have escaped the surgeon's knife. By killing cells directly by ionizing radiation, radiotherapy provides maximum protection and a guarantee against relapse in the future. The absence of cancer cells in the lymph nodes in Carol's case meant that she was spared a course of chemotherapy, more toxic and aggressive to the body than radiotherapy. She was also prescribed Tamoxifen for 5 years as a standard procedure. This is a hormone therapy that blocks estrogens, which have a well-known role in the genesis of breast cancers.

As all the results of her check-ups come back negative, Carol is considered cured.

The situation deteriorates

Barely 18 months later, in October, 1999, Carol complains of pain in the liver area. She has her blood tests done, which reveal that her cancer has returned with a vengeance. Her tumor markers of breast cancer, known as CA 15/3, have reached 770 units, where the normal level should be less than 31! An urgent scan was ordered that shows up multiple metastases in the liver, each up to 2 centimeters in diameter. The radiologist's report said, "there were too many to be counted."

Extremely shocked by this finding, the cancer specialists are at a loss to understand why the hormone treatment had been so ineffectual. They collectively decide to stop the Tamoxifen and immediately institute a course of high-dose chemotherapy, to be administered over the following six months.

Carol embarks on this new treatment with courage and full of hope. The first review after three months, in February, 2000, shows a slight decrease in the size of the tumors.

The metastases are gaining ground

However, only a month later, complaining of pain in the left side of her ribcage, she is given a PET scan in order to evaluate the activity of cancer cells. It shows that the cancer has spread to her bones, and also there has been a significant worsening of the metastases in the liver in such a short time. In a state of panic, Carol dreads that nothing can hold back the progress of this terrible disease in her body.

Her oncologists decide to have her undergo local radiotherapy, targeted on the ribs infiltrated by cancer, although this area had already been irradiated during the first radiation session to the breast and thorax. They are desperate to try everything to save Carol and make use all of the weapons at their disposal. So, they decide to start her on a new type of anti-hormonal treatment.

A new hope arises in France

Despite taking the new drug treatments conscientiously for nine months, in early 2001, one of the metastases in her liver was found to have grown considerably and Carol begins to feel that she is losing the battle. She knows that she will have to look in other quarters if she is to survive. It so happened that she met Angela R during an Avon three-day Breast Cancer Walk she had joined. This marks a turning point in her search. Angela, who was suffering from metastatic endometrial cancer, recommended she see the French doctor who is treating her in Paris in close collaboration with her surgeon in Los Angeles. Her American physician had to admit that the two types of treatment had worked very well together because the patient had been cured.

Angela's enthusiasm gave Carol some hope and she decides to come to Paris to see me.

Carol's first visit to my office in Paris

Before coming to Paris, Carol had sent me her file. By that time, her breast cancer had been first identified 3 years previously, and then had metastasized to her liver and bones 18 months later.

Her file was bulky and put together remarkably well, as American doctors certainly know how. Her medical records highlight the difficulties faced by doctors when they come up against these stubborn cases that fail to respond to even the most powerful treatments. I could see that Carol's physicians had treated her as well as they possibly could, with all the latest therapeutic techniques at their disposal. What should we think about all this? As you can imagine, a lot of questions came to mind, for myself and for the sake of the patient.

How can it be that a woman treated by the most respected American specialists in gynecology, surgery, endocrinology, radiotherapy, and oncology could relapse so quickly after the most effective medical treatments available anywhere? How, in the first place, can a woman in excellent health, with a healthy lifestyle, suddenly develop an apparently treatable breast cancer when she had been only taking menopausal HRT for a few months? How could it have invaded her liver and bones in less than 2 years?

In my practice, I have often seen patients with life-threatening illness. What do you say to a patient whose cancer no longer responds to the most advanced treatments that research can offer? When they say: "Doctor, I am worried, my treatment no longer seems to be working. My markers keep going up. My scan shows new lesions, the X-ray of my lungs doesn't look good, my backache is getting worse, and I am very scared. Tell me: are you going to save my life? I know that I should continue to fight, but I can no longer stand your chemo with the constant vomiting and diarrhea, I have lost so much weight and am so dizzy, I can barely stand, ask my husband … and still my test results get worse each month in spite of the treatment. Tell me, Doctor, how bad is it? Am I going to die?"

Doctors strive to treat their cancer patients to the best of their abilities, using science and best practice and following all the treatment protocols. All these measures usually work very quickly, even though the side effects take a heavy toll. Unfortunately, there are cases where the strongest weapons seem to be losing their power and fail to prevent the disastrous progression or relapses. In such cases, we are at a loss what else to know do. How to interpret these situations and how to answer patient's questions, pain, fears, and hopes? The doctor comes up against the limits of his or her knowledge and convictions and has to face uncertainties and difficult choices.

Is this not the time to broaden horizons, and adopt a broader approach to the patient? Rather than seeing the patient just through their cancer, wouldn't it be better to see him or her as a whole, as a unique being? Why should we deprive ourselves of a new outlook, of a different perspective than that which is currently in vogue and which focuses mainly on the disease? Is there not a medical approach that would allow us to understand the mechanisms by which cancerous cells were not only able to circumvent the effects of chemotherapy and hormonal treatment but, in Carol's case, were able to grow and disseminate in her body with such rapidity that in a few months her cancer had reached stage 4? Stage 4 is the last stage where the chances of survival, even for a short time, are very low.

Carol comes to Paris and here she is, standing in my office. The first thing that strikes me is the way she looks at me. Her eyes bore into mine as if to guess the depth of my thinking, leaving me no place to hide. She wants to get down to business.

Her twin sister accompanies her, unwavering in her support. They have the same smile, and the same determination to live, coupled with an unflinching desire to be told how things really stand, no matter how painful the truth might be. In a frank and open dialog, we assess her situation, point by point. She knows full well the severity of her condition and if she decided to come to Paris, despite the distance and the fatigue of travel, it is because she is determined to try everything, providing it is reasonable and plausible. Her trust in me did not falter and was deepened by the continuity of our communication, through consultations and the exchange of emails. Carol's confidence is strengthened by her knowing that I had worked for 7 years in an oncology hospital in Paris, and that I would not embark on any treatment without first informing her American oncologist and receiving his consent.

She never at any point gave up her fight against the disease. I did not know back then that her fight was going to last so many years with so many pitfalls to overcome, but in the end we managed to stabilize her condition for over 9 years. Carol is eager to know everything about her case because, as she says, that is the only way she can actually deal with it: how can we fight without understanding our adversary? It is not easy to remain visibly unmoved when seeing a patient with such an advanced stage of cancer. As with any disease, the first thing to do when seeing a patient is to listen.

The history of her disease provides a mass of information: the cancer, the way it first appeared, its type and its histology, the tests, the reports, the findings, and so on. But is this really helpful? How are you going to find the minute details about those imbalances which, millimeter by millimeter, day after day, over the years, led Carol via a long pathway of incubation, to her cancer and to its rapid growth and its alarming spread throughout her body?

Carol has come to understand that her current state had not been the consequence of chance alone, as if to say "You are one of the unfortunate cases." The conventional view sees bad luck as one of the "causes" but now Carol knows better.

Cancer doesn't happen by chance

But chance has no place in the human body; it is a word we physicians use to hide our failures of discernment and acknowledge that our understanding of the complexity of living beings is limited. The ineluctable chain of physiological events that lead from abnormalities in a single cell to the development of cancer, and then to widespread cancer, are complex and difficult to understand. But that should not deter us from trying to identify them. However, this process takes time and it is very difficult to fit in with the current medical approach to cancer, where time is constrained with too many and too few practitioners, and so everything is always is rushed. These and other factors make it nigh impossible to adopt a broad and more considered approach to the cancer patient.

A completely new methodology is needed if we are to develop a rational approach to treatment that takes into account the sick person in his or her totality. Such methods would enable true preventative work and provide support people through their illness and treatment.

The entirety of the patient's life is involved in the expression of his or her cancer, and so you cannot reach a true understanding of this disease if you limit yourself to the narrow study of the usual culprits: diet, tobacco, pollution, endocrine disruptors, and the like. It is essential to go deeper: to position the disease within the structure of the individual, to understand how their structure very gradually became out of kilter. You need to find out how they adapted to the cumulative challenges of life, whatever they happened to be, and whether their protective systems were induced to give up the struggle gradually or abruptly.

In Carol's case, there are some clear indications that the disease had its origins at a much earlier time than the appearance of the tumor. It is a mistake to think that cancer struck suddenly.

The root causes of the disease

It was obvious that several related factors played a large role in the emergence of cancer in this remarkable woman. Tracing the details of Carol's history, as a private detective might, represents a crucial first step. Looking for these clues will allow us to better understand the genesis of her disease.

Some elements that increased the chances of cancer were rooted in the structure of Carol's body. While we all have the same generic human structure, each of us has a different ability to use the energy the body needs to function and to deal with the challenges that life throws at us. There are human beings who are born with a slow thyroid and who will consequently need a great deal of sleep, while others who are constitutionally hyperactive and sleep little because they have a very active thyroid. Similarly, some are able to work a lot without feeling fatigue, because their adrenal gland is very active, while others whose adrenal is less active become tired after little effort. This personal level of functioning is *specific to everyone*, and does not at all suggest that there is any specific disease of either the thyroid or the adrenal glands. The potential of the individual can only be expressed according to his or her own capacities.

There are different types of structures. How they variously react and respond to the world gives us an insight into the very different pathway that the same cancer, of the breast, or the thyroid for example, will take in two different people. How it develops, where it is exactly sited, how it will respond to treatment, is characteristic and specific to the person's initial structure, as are the organs implicated in the genesis of the disease. Some women will develop breast cancer that will be permanently cured by a simple surgical intervention, while others, having an apparently identical cancer, will go from bad to worse. But why?

The keys to understanding

One of the key points we need to understand is that our body (the structure) operates in a very particular way for each person. It is governed by hormones that, acting at all times at all levels of our being, regulate the performance of the organs. It is these that allow us to survive and thrive. The hormones ensure the functioning, regulation, repair, and protection of each organ and of the body as a whole.

This is why, to properly and accurately assess any patient suffering from any kind of cancer, it is vital to make a full evaluation of the state of the entire hormonal system, and to study, in parallel, the organs' response to the action exerted by the hormonal system. The risk of developing breast cancer is not the same in everyone but depends on the hormonal activity of each woman. The fact of having high levels of female hormones is not of itself a great risk, but if these estrogens are also metabolically very active, the risk increases especially where this excess is coupled with other factors that accentuate the risk.

For example, a very active thyroid gland will act as an accelerator. In Carol's case, estrogens were constitutionally very active. In addition, the activity of her androgens (male hormones, secreted by the ovary) was also high. It was this combination that increased her potential risk of initiating cancer one day.

The high level of activity of these two types of hormones could also be evaluated, not only by studying the entire history of her life, but also through specific morphological traits (her general appearance, body fat distribution, etc.), and by knowing the various illness to which she had previously succumbed, as well as by analyzing her personality.

Her hormonal structure bequeathed her a vigorous temperament with the ability to manage a business and to assume important responsibilities. This strong character worked against her, as the professional difficulties she encountered led to excessive effort and drove her to the point of exhaustion, and thus contributed to weaken her resistance to illness. Because Carol has never been able to listen to her body and let go, her "never give up" character pushed her to exceed her limits and get extremely tired, which raised her stress level and caused the emergence her illness and, later, its intensification.

It had often been thought, and is now proven, that hormones not only carve our morphology and control our entire metabolism, but they act deeply on our character, our emotional life, our dreams, and our imagination. Numerous studies have demonstrated that they shape our behavior. It has been shown, for example, that the maternal attitude of mothers who have given birth develops in direct relationship with her levels of prolactin, the hormone that stimulates the production of milk. This is an adaptation mechanism, which ensures the infant will receive both nutrition and protection. Similarly, oxytocin, produced by the pituitary gland, and sometimes known as the love hormone, plays a major role in positive behavior: trust, love, and fidelity. Other studies have also shown that people with autism have an oxytocin deficiency, which may explain, in part, their difficulty to communicate with others.

However, the influence of hormones on behavior can be seen not only in extreme cases of dysfunction where their effects are obvious, but also in everyone's daily life, in very subtle ways. We must pay the utmost attention to all the clues given by the patient to be able to properly assess the role played by a hormone in the emergence of a sign. Generally, a balanced and nuanced overall hormonal state contributes to our personality. There are, by contrast, specific hormonal pathologies (often an excessive thyroid function) that give rise to extreme behaviors like, for example, manic episodes.

This entire enquiry will require the doctor to devote a great deal of time to each and every patient. The human body is perpetually changing and participates in a world that acts upon it constantly, and so its signs are also evolving, and reflect the transformations within. This is why we take a comprehensive medical approach, and one that Carol came to appreciate. It consists of following very carefully any change in the signs and symptoms, the better to understand the patient's state.

All physicians would agree that real medicine involves listening, touching, analyzing, adapting the treatment, and permanently questioning the results. In the twenty-first century, we are able to practice personalized medicine and not an impersonal medicine of statistical individuals. Our patients deserve nothing less.

To return to Carol's case, in addition to her potentially dangerous structural characteristics, the internal strife as much as external aggressors that she had experienced in various ways further increased her risk of developing cancer.

First, stress

Faced with professional difficulties, Carol had to take on a great deal of responsibility and many commitments to meet. She mobilized her entire being to this end, and this strain triggered, at the level, a deep and permanent activation of her alert systems to provide the necessary surplus of energy, with grave consequences. Any significant change in lifestyle, any major new and unexpected aggression, physical or mental, inevitably requires a physiological response and calls upon very precise changes from the body. Emotional shock in anyone is always followed by a bodily reaction. Stress is not only in the head, but also at the same time in the body because it is the physiological response to the aggression.

There is a widespread popular misconception about stress that often reduces it to emotional stress, focusing exclusively on the psychological aspect. We say: "I am stressed," "I have too much stress." Stress is certainly something we feel: anxiety, fear, restlessness, self-doubt, but the immediate reaction to a situation is primarily a physical one and involves the alert system with a discharge of adrenaline and the release of glucose from the liver to provide immediate energy. Stress involves complex mechanisms and is more intricate than simple distress. Along with emotional feelings, a cascade of physiological reactions is triggered in the body to muster all available resources to deal with the aggression.

This mobilization demands a lot of energy and, depending on the state of the patient at the time, may induce or exacerbate disease. Merely prescribing tranquilizers or antidepressants to the stressed or depressed individual is a niggardly medical response to what in reality is a highly complex situation. The lack of attention paid to the body by a simplistic psychological approach, as if stress causes only mental suffering, is an unfortunate consequence of the kind of compartmentalized medical thinking that patients complain about. A genuinely integrative approach must try to consider everything that happens in the body at the time that the patient experienced the shock.

In Carol's case, because her stress was excessive and went on for a long time and therefore involved her whole being as well as various organs and bodily functions that were already out of balance, she should not have been treated solely with antidepressants and sedatives. Rather she should have been offered comprehensive support, integrating her psychological feelings with physiological change. In the absence of a broad approach to treatment, her structural hormonal imbalances deteriorated and culminated in various physiological patterns becoming entrenched, which included the over-solicitation of her already malfunctioning thyroid gland, a demand on insulin to provide energy, and congestion of her liver from her overactive of sympathetic nervous system. This chain of disturbances led inevitably to disease.

When stress becomes chronic and weakens immunity

The need to constantly cope with a difficult professional situation over a long period of time generated a state of chronic stress in Carol and absorbed all her energy. Many studies have shown that hormones like ACTH and cortisol which are secreted during such states cumulatively block cell-mediated immunity, acting particularly on the thymus gland which plays an important role in the synthesis of antibodies. The progressive weakening of her immune system would have been a combined risk factor with the strong estrogen pressure on all the cells of her body. Subjected to this constant aggression, Carol's body behaves a bit like a compass with the needle forever spinning without ever returning to its initial position. Her body is going to have to adapt during this

critical period. For her to remain healthy it will have to do so in a positive manner.

During the menopause, a woman's terrain becomes vulnerable to the
emergence of serious problems. Carol is thus at a critical stage, and is
associated with a high level of risk. This explosive situation needs only
a detonator to set if off.

The menopause: the detonator

The final blow was delivered by the inappropriate prescription of hormone replacement therapy. The pill contained both estrogen and progesterone. These are the female hormones that the body produces in
the second half of the normal menstrual cycle; their natural function in
the event of fertilization is to protect early pregnancy. But Carol already
had an overabundance of female hormones in her body, given her own
structure and compounded by her dietary regime. Her gynecologist
prescribed her this treatment without in any way assessing her hormonal status. This is currently how millions of women are treated. As
the treatment created a hormonal overload at the critical onset of the
menopause, is it not unreasonable to suggest, with hindsight, that it
acted as a catalyst in the formation of the tumor, or its growth if it was
already present but too small to be seen on a mammogram.

The speed with which the tumor appeared was the *tip of the iceberg*,
indicating the deep imbalances that had been building up gradually,
over the months and years, hidden in the recesses of her body's metabolism. Carol's entire life was enclosed within her breast, and the different
stages of her life were transcribed into her cancer.

The biological analyses fully endorsed the validity of these conclusions. The biopsies taken from Carol's breast tumor showed that the
cancer cells contained a large number of estrogen and progesterone
receptors. This strongly suggests that the HRT played an important participatory role in her case, but cannot be the complete explanation as
many women take such hormone treatments, and do not go on to develop
breast cancer! But hormone replacement therapy was potentially dangerous for Carol's particular terrain, and performed the role of detonator.

Diet: the burden we impose on our bodies

Her terrain was all the more at risk because she had been on a strict
vegetarian diet for more than 10 years and it was one in which soybeans

predominated. While such a diet cannot cause cancer on its own, in a terrain that was already overloaded with estrogen, as was the case with Carol, it would certainly be a risk factor in adding further to this excess. Studies have shown the soybean to be very rich in phytoestrogens, which have an effect on the body similar to that of estrogen, which proved harmful in her particular case.

Carol's biology of functions

Carol arrived with the results of a CT scan that had been done a week before her visit. By using X-rays to produce cross-sectional views of the body, it showed that a new lesion was developing in her liver. She also brought results from a lab test done just before she left for France.

The algorithm in the Biology of Functions will use these lab tests to calculate her indexes. We will rerun further tests at each consultation, from which we will generate a graph so that we can chart her progress. This gives us the opportunity to assess the changes in the state of her body as we proceed with treatments and follow-up her case. In her autobiographical book, Carol has detailed at length the changes in her blood test results and how the corresponding indexes evolved over time, allowing you to see the patient from another angle.

This first integrative biology, which will be followed by many others, gives an overall view of the structure of her body, and also shows how it manages to adapt to different circumstances. It shows very clearly how Carol is drowning in a veritable sea of estrogen with an activity three to four times higher than normal. Her follicular index is very high, too, which is an aggravating factor: one of the effects of follicle stimulating hormone (FSH) is to increase the number of estrogen receptors and thus fuel the development of cancer.

The situation is even more critical, as the corticotropic axis, which plays a major role in the distribution of energy substrates needed for the normal functioning of metabolism, is in an advanced pathological state. The histamine index, which explores part of the activity of this axis, is also high, which means there is a considerable amount of congestion in those areas where estrogens are concentrated, particularly in the liver. All of this is consistent with the spread of metastases throughout her body. In addition, her prolactin index is very high, indicating excessive production of both androgens and estrogens, which are already overloading Carol's body. Most of the indexes that deal directly with cancerous disease itself are, as you might expect, in the red. The adenosis index, which describes the level of hormonal elements fueling her tumors, is considerably active, as are the growth factors, which stimulate the development of pathological cells.

The indexes which reflect the degree of cell damage and ruptures in the integrity of DNA were extremely high. These results came as no surprise, unwelcome as they were; they testified to the intensity of the fire within her that was raging out of control.

All was not lost, however. There were some positive factors in her favor which would help her fight this disease: the metabolic activity of the thyroid has remained relatively low, which explains why Carol put on 10 kilos since her diagnosis; in spite of several diets and sporting activities, she was unable to lose any weight. Fortunately, this relative weakness of her thyroid increases her insulin resistance, and so restricts the entry of nutrients into cancerous cells, which have a higher need than normal cells. Still, Carol tires quickly. Although her adrenal gland is fighting valiantly, the high levels of cortisol that are trying to quench the huge inflammation invading her body, the hormone that stimulates cortisol production (known as ACTH), cannot respond to this level of demand for ever.

The breakdown of hormonal equilibrium explains the rapidity with which the metastases are forming and spreading. In spite of this highly dangerous situation, some other indexes are fortunately still favorable. Apoptosis, the process that persuades diseased cells to die, generally declines with cancer, but in her case the index shows quite the opposite. Likewise, her anti-growth factors are very high. These are factors that resist the growth of tumors, against growth factors that stimulate them. These rare pieces of good news tell us that Carol still has a slim but realistic chance of beating the disease in the long-term. Provided, of course, that she is given the support to do so.

Clearly this support should not be a repeat of the treatment she had previously been given as it had failed to slow down the development of her cancer. Her Biology of Functions is nothing short of disastrous: the imbalances and the paradoxical findings in Carol's body are so complex, that we need to design a highly specific physiological treatment, if we are to have any hope of helping her. Precise diagnoses cannot be matched up with standardized treatments, prescribed blindly or formulated on a one-size-fits-all approach. To make fully informed therapeutic decisions you need to understand fully the nature of that which you are trying to address. Personalized prescribing is imperative if we are to avoid the disastrous consequences of the standardization which puts vulnerable people at even greater risk.

After our lengthy consultation, a new understanding of Carol's state has emerged thanks to our simultaneous consideration of the disease, the sick person, the current treatment, and the relations between these different elements. This will give us an insight into the deep-seated causes of her body's failure to respond previously to powerful treatments and will enable us to formulate a new therapeutic plan and give her the best means of protecting herself.

The treatment will be personalized and will aim at restoring the balance in her body. We must try to prevent the emergence of new metastases and stabilize the old tumors. I sent a report to Carol's oncologist in the States to keep him informed about the diagnosis and treatment. I suggested, if he agreed, that we stop the Mégace immediately. This is a hormonal therapy based on progesterone and her body is already saturated with estrogen and progesterone. Besides, it had failed to prevent the rapid increase of the tumors in the liver, and anyway standard practice reserves it for the breast cancer. This is not to say that this drug is ineffective, but its efficacy depends upon an accurate diagnosis.

The aim of endobiogenic treatment

Based on the diagnostic conclusions, the Endobiogenic treatment will aim to provide support for Carol's whole body. As for the cancer, we will try to work with her oncologist towards the elimination of the tumors but with a more targeted approach than taken previously. Our priority will aim to correct the imbalances in Carol's body, which are contributing directly or indirectly to the progression of her illness.

The strategy will attempt the following:

- to reduce the production and supply of elements that feed the cancer cells;
- to stimulate her immune and hormonal functions to slow down tumor growth;
- to support her body in its fight against the disease and to minimize the side effects from chemotherapy;
- to clean up the mess created by the various remedies given her previously and which continue to overburden the remaining healthy cells in her liver.

This first treatment provides gentle drainage, supporting an exhausted body from months of fighting the disease, and aims to reduce the intensity of the pelvic and hepatic congestion found on clinical examination. Restoring the balance of her autonomic nervous system will be one of the first areas to be addressed as it played such an important part in the development of her illness, and is still much too active, especially her alpha-sympathetic system. The major therapeutic goals will be to reduce the over-production of the sex hormones, to regulate her thyroid axis and so help with energy supply, and to reduce the growth factors which favor the growth of cancer.

We will look to natural-based products, mainly medicinal plants to obtain these benefits, according to the methods outlined in Chapter 6. I am well disposed to the resumption of chemotherapy to kill the cancer cells, providing it is administered in conjunction with the treatments that I have prescribed to treat the problems underlying the cancer. When I worked in the Oncology Department at Boucicaut Hospital, I saw too many patients die very quickly from the toxic load of chemotherapy that their already depleted bodies could not withstand.

My practice of medicine over the last 40 years has persuaded me that had all patients been supported in their struggle with disease by treatments customized to their own particular state quite a few of them would have fared better. A growing number of contemporary works, particularly in the United States, attest to the potential benefits of medicinal plants.

Targeted support with treatments based on medicinal plants

Only plants with well-documented and demonstrable effects can be selected for Carol's treatment and their use can only be justified by those with actions that are well matched to the changes we are trying to induce in her body.

The need to drain her body of the many toxins it has accumulated justifies the choice of blackcurrant leaves (*Ribes nigrum*), to help support her exhausted adrenal glands, and Chrysanthellum leaves (from a tropical species *Chrysanthellum americanum*), to ensure the proper functioning of her digestive system. To obtain such effects she will be asked to prepare a decoction of these two plants and drink a liter per day. These two plants provide the necessary background therapy needed to prepare the body for the whole-plant extracts of the medicinal plants that make up the rest of the prescription, as follows:

- Gromwell (*Lithospermum officinalis*)
  the whole plant, but especially the seeds
  to slow down the production of estrogens
- Sequoia (*Sequoia gigantea*)
  the buds
  to block the production of estrogens receptors in the liver, and to promote bone reconstruction after the metastatic events of February, 2000
- Salad burnet (*Poterium sanguisorba*)
  The root
  to slow down the activity of growth hormone
  and of prolactin, a hormone that stimulates the production of androgens and estrogens
- Gypsywort (*Lycopus europea*)
  the whole plant and
  Pichi (*Fabiana imbricata*), a shrub from Chile
  young branches
  to slow down the thyroid axis and the conversion of thyroxin (T4) into triiodothyronine (T3);
  these thyroid hormones speed up energy metabolism and stimulate cell growth
- Oak (*Quercus pedunculata*)
  the *buds*
  to promote pelvic decongestion by venous stimulation, and favor the reconstruction bone by osteoblasts (these are cells responsible for the formation of bone matrix)
- Chaste tree (*Vitex agnus castus*)
  leaves and fruit
  to reduce estrogenic hyperactivity
  to restore the balance of the autonomic nervous system, by reducing alpha-sympathetic hyperactivity
- Mistletoe (*Viscum album*)
  whole-plant extract
  to stimulate her immune system
- Vitamin C and magnesium to decrease her high level of oxidation and revitalize her body.

Personalized nutrition for a patient with cancer

Dietary advice is an important feature in the treatment of cancer. Given Carol's case history, she would be well advised to stop eating the following foods:

— All forms of sugar, because they stimulate the secretion of insulin which contributes to cellular nutrition, and cancer cells in particular: they can consume their weight in glucose every four to five hours;
— Dairy products, because they contain proteins which tend to promote the inflammatory state and the production of immunoglobulins in the small intestine, are a source of allergies. They also contain cholesterol, which is a precursor of estrogens;
— Soybeans, because they contain phyto-estrogens and may be counterproductive in her hyper-estrogenic state;
— Cereals like wheat, because they can also stimulate the production of immunoglobulins, a potential source of an allergic response.

Carol is an extrovert and likes to party and so asks me if she can drink wine. I tell her that given the current state of her liver, she should abstain totally for the present. In time she could enjoy the occasional glass of red wine with its putative benefits (but never more than one glass a day) but I advise her to exclude white wine completely. I suggest she pay no attention to standard dietary advice in books and magazines, which doesn't cater for the individual, completely and can even in some cases, be harmful.

Research has shown that women who have a twin sister with breast cancer are four times more likely to develop the same disease and so Carol asks me to do a biological assessment of her twin sister, Cheryl, who came with her and with whom she is very close. She wants me then to establish a personalized terrain-based treatment for her, striving to head off the threat of the disease with a truly preventative medical approach.

Six months later: second consultation

Carol reported that the Endobiogenic treatment had greatly helped her: with energy levels back to normal, and she no longer had the intense stomach pain. Her oncologist had replaced the Mégace with Xeloda an oral chemotherapy protocol with less harsh side effects: confined to irritation in the palms of the hands and soles of the feet, and diarrhea, but at least no loss of hair.

The treatments had aimed to restore equilibrium in her body, and thereby raise her tolerance to chemotherapy. Her recent blood test results confirm that her general condition has improved significantly, with several indexes moving in a favorable direction. They indicate that her body is mobilizing itself to fight this cancer. Tumor markers are down by 9 points, estrogens have decreased by 25%, the carcinogenesis index has dropped considerably: from 173 to 18 (normal range 1 to 3); the involvement of the thyroid gland in the development of the disease has been reduced by 40%, while the anti-growth factors have increased. The hope of being able to achieve some measure of control begins to stir.

Carol's sister, Cheryl, came with her and brought the results of her own blood tests. According to these, her body is saturated with antioxidants, so she would be advised to stop taking all her vitamins and antioxidants immediately as they can have negative consequences in the long run. This uncontrolled self-medication is a fact of life in the United States, and becoming so in France, a trend encouraged by some laboratories, with their sights on huge over-the-counter sales. I worry about the overconsumption of these products that are peddled indiscriminately as if they are beneficial for everyone's health. They conceal potential adverse effects, which may lie dormant in the body for a long while before initiating a disorder.

We should treat all medicinal products with respect and take them with due caution, not just powerful synthetic drugs, but also these over-the-counter products, especially plant extracts, vitamins, antioxidants, and other so-called natural substances: they all have an impact on the human body.

Six months later: third consultation

The physiological data concerning Carol's terrain continues to improve. The results from her blood tests remain good, but the data provided by the Biology of Functions are a very different story. All of a sudden, the stress indexes have risen dangerously, and at this rate is likely to jeopardize before long all the progress we have made.

The cortico-adrenal index, which gives an idea of the intensity of stress experienced by the body, has jumped to four times the normal level. The activity of the hormone ACTH, which stimulates the adrenal glands, has gone up from 12 to 472 (the normal range being between 0.7 and 3) indicating that Carol is under huge stress. The index of DHEA, an androgen produced in the adrenal gland, has shot up from 24 to 3,248. This is especially concerning because this hormone can be converted to estrogen and so risks reenergizing the tumors. All these elements herald a likely relapse of cancer.

I am very worried about this abrupt reversal of her internal milieu and wonder what new circumstances can explain such a remarkable increase. What injurious events in Carol's life are mirrored in her body with an intensity that may turn against her, unless we take steps to diminish them? She explains she is struggling to cope with huge commercial pressures that threaten the very survival of her business and she has to cope with it all single-handedly. While this explains why her results are so much worse, I have to point out that this level of stress can have a devastating effect on the development of cancer. Stress triggers a very complex reaction in the body, known as the "general adaptation syndrome." This stimulates the metabolic and endocrine systems in order to provide the energy the body will need to deal with the aggressor, whether external or from within. Cancer cells can capture and use this available energy for their own growth. At the same time, the stress tends to weaken the immune system, which is already under pressure to fight the cancer cells.

The stakes are very high. Carol has two choices, either she continues to wear herself out, while in a very advanced stage of cancer, or she takes my advice and gives up her business. The choice facing her is as clear as it is difficult, but in the end unavoidable. We often need to know how to win by losing, especially when life is at stake. Carol will have to find a way to reduce her work pressures by selling her company outright or by finding an investor to take over her responsibilities.

When writing the prescriptions for the next phase of treatment I shall have to consider this new risk factor of elevated stress. It is vital to inhibit the secretion of ACTH and the conversion of DHEA into estrogen.

Six months later: fourth consultation

Carol decided to follow my advice and sell her company, which had been the cause of her stress in the first place. The sale continues to make her extremely anxious and it will take a year for it all to be settled and for her to be freed from a state of continual worry. Reading the latest blood tests make me uneasy about her prospects. We are now at the start of the fall; in common with spring, this is a time of important hormonal transition. Adaptation to seasonal change involves the endocrine system and so makes chronic disease more susceptible to relapse. There are signs that Carol's cancer is gaining ground: her estrogens are on the rise again, kept high by a surge in prolactin. The *turnover* index is up again, a sign of poor cellular repair and renewal. Indexes of carcinogenesis and growth factors are rising, as is histamine, which is involved in the inflammatory response. These indexes offer a window on the working of the terrain and allow us to predict the future development of the disease. The standard tumor marker, by contrast, can only give a snapshot of the current level of activity of her cancer and is unable to anticipate future developments. Hers has continued to come down, and at 20.5 would seem to show an improving trend, but this is a deceptive sign.

Listening to these explanations, Carol remembers that it was in the fall 2 years previously that her breast cancer had been discovered, followed by metastasis into her liver. The recent stress has had the effect of returning Carol's body back to the place where it had been 18 months before. The stress has delayed her body's move towards balance, but has not prevented it. All it needed now was more time to restore the equilibrium, now that the business problem had been solved.

Six months later: fifth consultation

Carol had got to know her body better, to understand her reactions and to appreciate how diet or stress can upset its balance. My approach differs from that of her American physician who is focused on the tumors in her liver while my aim is to balance her body in its entirety, not just her liver. But Carol is alarmed: her oncologist in the United States gave her 2 years to live, and that was 3.5 years ago! Carol is agonizing over how long she has to live. I urge her to give up this survival mentality and free herself from fear. I reassure her that in spite of the tumors that have invaded her liver, her new overall equilibrium is compatible with many years of life.

These regular blood tests allow us to see subtle changes in her body and, therefore, to anticipate any beneficial or adverse trends. They give me the opportunity to modify and adapt her treatment accordingly. Carol is worried about a small rise in her tumor marker, CA 15/3, to slightly above the normal range. I point out that the great majority of the Biology of Functions indexes are significantly improved. The negative effects of stress no longer have the same intense effect on her body and she is now back on course towards a new point of equilibrium. I am also able to reassure her that fluctuations of tumor markers are fairly typical, and as long as they remain close to the normal range, even if a little high she has no need to be unduly worried. I suggest she practice yoga to calm her mind and to raise her spirits and to see an osteopath to help her maintain better physical equilibrium.

We fortify her treatment with seven new medicines, which aim to revitalize her body, reduce congestion, and support the eliminative functions of her liver and kidney. Several therapies are prescribed for drainage:

- A 21-day course of whole lemon therapy, once every two months, to improve the fluidity of the blood and reduce the risk of vascular disorders.
- A ten-day course of melon therapy, once every two months, for its diuretic effects. Three introductory days (brown rice the first day, vegetables the second, fruit the third), are followed by four days of melon only, and then three closing days in the reverse order to the introductory days, finishing with brown rice only on the final day.
- A ten-day pineapple cure, once every two months, alternating with the melon cure, as a method of fat reduction.

Carol tells me later that she feels the weight of the world has been lifted off her shoulders. She is free of her fears about how much longer she has left to live and is starting to replace the survival mode with a sense of serenity about her future.

Six months later: sixth consultation

Stress now belongs to the past. Almost all her indexes are significantly better than those she brought to her first consultation. I would say that Carol's body has reached a point of equilibrium as never before. For the first time, Carol, whom her doctors gave only a 3% chance of survival, no longer feels that she is in imminent danger. She is still under a chemotherapy regime (Xeloda), which she tolerates very well.

In May, 2004, 4.5 years after multiple metastases were found in her liver, Carol's health is as good as she can hope for at this stage. She not only feels well, but as a testament to her experiences she has decided to write a book to describe the path she has taken. Her determination to spread the word that cancer, even when very advanced, need not be a cause for despair, spurs her on to write the book in less than a year. She is on a mission to tell others about the rational treatments that can be taken alongside conventional chemotherapy, even in cases that are considered hopeless.

The book became an overnight success, and changed Carol's life dramatically. She became a living example for the many American women living with cancer. She made herself available at all hours of day or night, to encourage and explain how to live with generalized breast cancer and not lose hope, even when all seems lost.

She affirms tirelessly, going on television to explain that her cancer was not stabilized by a miracle, but followed an Endobiogenic assessment of her terrain with comprehensive treatments designed to restore her body to a more balanced state. She is convinced that anyone with cancer should be able to benefit from the considerable help offered by the Endobiogenic approach, as a complement to chemotherapy or radiotherapy.

Living 10 years with cancer

Over the years Carol and I kept up our regular consultations, during which I followed-up her case very closely either through the internet or at training seminars that I conducted in the United States, in which she often took part. But the vagaries of life and the burden of her conventional treatments took their toll. Her tumors, progressively failing to respond to chemotherapy, little by little overwhelmed her. In spite of more intense Endobiogenic treatment, Carol's body continued to weaken, and the cancer markers rose again. The more the chemotherapy was intensified, the more the disease seemed to evade any attempt to curb it.

The year 2008 turned out to be a very difficult one. Aware that the last stage of her life was getting closer, I decided to visit her at her home in Santa Barbara. On a sunny day in June and surrounded by those close to her, Carol looked radiant. In deference to all who had come, she asked to be helped out of her bed, that she had not left for some days, to sit on an armchair that had been set up on the terrace of the house, which looked out over a large valley. Attentive to all, she shares her last counsel with each one. She has prepared her leaving very carefully as she knows it is near, and expresses her love to everyone. Then she asks to speak to me alone and says a few words that will forever be engraved in my memory.

A few days later, on June 27, 2008, Carol leaves this life in a state of profound peace, as all those around her will testify.

An encouragement for those suffering from cancer

Carol's battle against cancer had taken her on a long journey during which she was able to lead a normal life for almost 9 years, even though the cancer had spread to her liver and bones. She came to appreciate how important it is to take an active role in the choice of treatments for the disease, and what a difference a truly integrative approach makes, taking into account the totality of the individual. She fully realized the point at which stress is detrimental to health, especially when the terrain has been weakened by disease, and how crucial it is to maintain body, mind, and spirit in equilibrium.

Regaining this equilibrium and maintaining it allows one to live with cancer, as with a chronic disease, keeping a watchful eye on it. Carol would often say that we live in a society marked by fear. This fear is transformed into intense anxiety when it comes to cancer. This grabs sufferers by the throat and prevents them from moving forward. Carol learned how to let go of it and replace it with hope. She wrote in her book: "if we can remain positive and confident that we can get our disease under control, then the years that we have ahead of us will be much more fulfilling. The fact that I know I have cancer, but also that it is stabilized and I can live a full life, gives me great strength. I hope that others will learn to keep their bodies in equilibrium, so as to be able to live with their cancer as if it were any other chronic disease, and with hope instead of fear."

CHAPTER TEN

Cancer: a troubling phenomenon

The number of cancers continues to grow

The scourge of cancer marches on unabated and is all the more distressing as the disease strikes younger and younger people and if we have not ourselves been affected, most of us will know someone who has. We all dread it: in the collective and personal psyche it is the harbinger of distress, danger, suffering, and death.

According to data provided by the French Health Watch Institute (*Institut de veille sanitaire*), 357,000[1] cancers were diagnosed in France in 2010 (203,000 in men, and 154,000 in women). The number of deaths for the same year was over 84,000 in men and over 62,000 in women. The number of new cases has increased by more than 70% over the past 20 years, and that number is projected to double by 2030. In 2007, 727,720 cases of cancer of all types were treated in France.[2]

In 2010, breast cancer still remains the commonest cancer in women with over 52,500 projected new cases of whom nearly 11,300 are expected to die. The disease is now discovered at a much younger age. It is projected that about 10,300 women, aged 15 to 49 years, will be diagnosed with breast cancer, as compared with 20 years ago when the number of young women suffering from it was lower and even less would their grandmother have been expected to suffer from it. Is this trend for the disease to affect younger age groups due to some environmental cause as our civilization creates more and more endocrine disruptors? (See Chapter 8 and Appendix 1). Some environmental contaminants (from agricultural and medicinal products, and many other pollutants) are already known while others no doubt wait to be identified.

Men do not escape cancer, either. There has been a veritable explosion in the number of prostate cancers. The annual number of new patients has doubled in less than 20 years: an estimate for 2010 predicted 71,500 new cases. Since this cancer, like that of the breast, is related to a dysregulation of the endocrine system, is it fair to assume that the origin of both these diseases, lies with the harm caused by endocrine disruptors?[3]

Colorectal cancer is the third most commonly cancer diagnosed in men (21,000 new cases announced), and the second in women (19,000 new cases). The much-feared lung cancer will affect some 27,000 men and 10,000 women with over 21,000 and 7,700 expected deaths respectively. In these cancers, life expectancy is very short: fewer than 15% of patients survive 5 years after diagnosis. Other cancers, such as lymphomas, melanomas, cancers of the thyroid, pancreas, bladder, and stomach are also showing an upward trend. Currently, health insurance covers 100% of the costs for more than 1,250,000 of our fellow citizens suffering from cancer, and the number of patients covered by the Long Term Illness Scheme[4] for cancer has increased by 62% in 10 years.

Faced with such an increase, we have to recognize that, unfortunately, in spite of all the research conducted towards understanding its causes and developing treatments, medical science has yet to come up with an explanation for this persistent rise in cancer. Nor has there been any improvement in prevention, or in a reduction in the rate of mortality.

Somehow the reality of the situation seems to have escaped those who argue that scientific progress will soon radically change the landscape. Such optimism fully expects that cancer will soon become a thing of the past, in the face of data that shows an opposite trend, one that serves to demonstrate that a purely analytical and reductive approach to cancer has been pushed to its limits. This approach is characterized by addressing the tumor itself, without taking into account the state of the patient in which it takes hold and grows.

A host of questions come to mind, some scientific, but also economic, industrial, political, and ethical questions, as we confront the fact that cancer is often resistant to very powerful treatments.

More and more expensive care

The cost of caring for cancers is huge and affects the healthcare budgets of every country. It has been estimated that the amount of money spent worldwide in 2010 exceeded $400 billion, nearly $20 billion in France (over €15 billion).

In addition to the costs incurred for screening, surgery, radiotherapy, and hospitalization, the costs of conventional chemotherapy amount to over $10 billion in seven of the major developed countries. In less than 10 years, the new so-called biological, or targeted products, have multiplied the costs of this class of treatment by a factor of six and have brought the manufacturers more than $20 billion in 2009, a figure that is expected to double in 5 years.[5] It is not difficult to understand the lucrative potential that any new molecule for combating cancer represents for those who develop it, and the legal, economic, and industrial conflicts that may arise. The manufacturer also needs to encourage doctors to prescribe their product, and so "expand its market," and increase the number of "consumers."

For example, Bevacizumab, which is manufactured by Roche Laboratories, ranks fourth among the most prescribed medicinal products in the world: 6.98 billion in 2010.[6] It is the leader in a new class of anticancer drugs, which have been hailed as a revolution in the treatment of cancer of the colon, breast, and bronchi. In 2008, based on promising results from trials on breast cancer, the FDA[7] placed this new bio-therapeutic molecule on "fast-track" (a procedure reserved for drugs that appear to promise real benefits in grave illness) and was given approval for the treatment of "metastatic breast cancer," which effectively guaranteed it huge sales. However, large-scale studies later showed that the expected benefits of this product did not outweigh its potential risks. When the FDA announced the withdrawal of its license, the pharmaceutical group Roche recruited groups of patients to testify in favor of keeping this product on the market, and lobbied hard to reverse the decision.[8] After consulting independent experts, and after a protracted legal battle, the FDA decided in December, 2010, that this medicinal product could no longer be licensed for the treatment of breast cancer, which stood to lose the company an estimated sum of more than $600 million in the United States alone.

Another example: on November 25, 2010, at the Second Meeting on Clinical Research held at Issy-les-Moulineaux, the German pharmaceutical group Bayer and the Norwegian pharmaceutical group Algeta announced that their anticancer drug Alpharadin, that had reached phase 3 in a clinical trial,[9] could improve the survival rate of patients with metastatic prostate cancer. The potential worldwide sales were estimated to reach $2 billion. On August 14, 2011, the FDA granted the priority review status for the fast-track approval of this product. The next day at the Frankfurt Stock Exchange, the value of the Algeta Group shares grew by 36%[10] even though the increase in life expectancy, which had been hailed as very promising, turned out to be a mere 2.8 months when compared with placebo! From a purely commercial point of view, the motives that fuel these belligerent legal campaigns are very clear.

What is cancer?

A brief life history of the normal cell

It is estimated that the human body is made up of 50 to 100 trillion cells, which are subdivided into 250 different cell types. They are all derived from the initial cell created at fertilization by the fusion of the father's sperm with the mother's egg. They all contain the same chromosomes as the initial cell, thus they all contain the same "library" of genes that determines both the structure and the functioning of the body, which provides the baseline for metabolism and the capacity to adapt. Each of us receives a unique legacy, which makes us unlike no other.

It is helpful to understand how a healthy cell works before considering how it can be transformed into a cancerous cell. The cell is considered the basic unit of life and can be thought of as a small factory of immense complexity. To operate, it needs material and energy such as glucose in the presence of oxygen, which is brought from the environment by the circulation according to its needs, and which will allow it to operate. It can then exercise its metabolic activity with two different but complementary purposes: either renew the various components of its structure, such as repairing its membrane, for example, or carry out some function for which it is programmed, such as making a protein or a hormone, and it must eliminate the waste generated by its work.

This factory is integrated within the larger system of the human body and is organized in a structured and coherent manner. The cell can survive only by maintaining close ties of with all the organs of the human body and all vital functions depend upon this continuous interdependence.

As trivial as it might sound, this basic concept has always to be kept in mind and will equip us for the task when faced with patients suffering from cancer. Today's oncologists tend to focus on eliminating pathological cells and consider the links connecting each cell with the entire body completely beside the point. Their approach focuses on the cancer itself and strives to destroy it at any price, by surgery, chemotherapy, and radiotherapy, the weapons of modern medicine. But these methods are not without their drawbacks: apart from the considerable toxicity of chemotherapy, the pace of the disease can outstrip the treatment and is prone to recur. Given the limitations of the current approach, is it not time to focus on the overall state of the individual in whom the cancerous cells have grown? Should we not take a broader approach that puts the person at the center of the management of their disease? It is time to enlarge this reductionist approach, which leaves the individual completely out of the picture.

All our cells communicate with one another

In the first eight weeks of intrauterine life, the fertilized cell develops into an embryo and then, with an exponential increase in complexity, the cells differentiate irreversibly and take on the specialized form and function that they will play throughout life: they commit themselves to the various tissues and organs that make up our body. The fate of each individual cell depends entirely upon the quality of the dialog it establishes with other cells in the community to which it belongs. Each of them transmits and receives complex molecular signals to and from their surface membranes and also to and from the cell's interior and nucleus. They also exchange small compounds and ions. The flow of messages from cell to cell both locally and, through the blood and lymphatic vessels and via the nervous system, at great distances, is constant and ceaseless. This incessant and complementary cooperation is vital, because it allows each cell to adapt in a very timely and precise manner to the size, architecture and functional state of every tissue and each organ to the needs of the whole human body.

This constructive cooperation allows them to manage all acute or chronic aggressions which come their way, and thus maintain the conditions essential to our life and health. The equilibrium and harmony of this immense community are made possible only by the hormonal system, this project manager, which regulates and coordinates all these relationships and thereby ensures the coherent and dependable functioning of the living being. If faulty information is established inside cells or between them, and if faulty cells escape central control, the door is wide open to the birth of cancer.

Each cell is specialized and designed for a specific purpose and cannot manufacture products indiscriminately: they can only produce what they are designed to do and can only operate according to software that is located inside their nucleus. This genetic program specifies the tasks to be performed. The genome is the entire genetic material of an individual person and each cell contains an identical copy and performs only the work assigned to it.[11] The scope and function of the cell is determined by the activation of the appropriate genes as it interacts with the demands of the environment. The switching on and off of genes is analogous to the choice of a software program even if a number of them are both installed on the hard drive of your computer, the one chosen will be that which is relevant to the task in hand.

So it is for our body. For example, the cells of the nervous system are programmed to process and transmit information, while those of the intestine are dedicated to the absorption of nutrients: proteins, carbohydrates, lipids, vitamins, and minerals. These cells have different functions, even though they share the same genome. They only use the program that had been assigned to them. In fact, once their function is assigned, they are unable to change it.

Only the undifferentiated cells—the so-called stem cells—have the capability of transforming themselves into any other cell by undergoing a process called differentiation. They cells are found in human embryos and can be collected from blood in the umbilical cord. They persist as adult stem cells, found in bone marrow; also in adipose tissue, and certain tissues in the nervous system. New techniques are being developed that permit the induction of a pluripotent state in cells derived from human skin. The creation of stem cells in the laboratory avoids having to use human embryos. They are the subject of an intense research effort. The objective of this cellular therapy is aimed at regenerating tissues or creating organs. However, because stem cells are so dynamic and can transform themselves very rapidly, they could potentially induce cancer or initiate a relapse, which makes their use much trickier than anticipated.

*Cells regenerate themselves throughout the life of the
human being*

Each cell has a certain life span, determined by the tissue to which it
belongs: a few hours for the cells of the gastrointestinal wall, a week for
the cornea of the eye, two weeks for skin cells, or four months for red
blood cells. Between successive divisions the cell enters into a phase
of the cell cycle known as interphase during which it cannot normally
divide and instead fulfills its normal function within the tissue or organ
in which it is located.

If the body is under pressure to renew some cells to repair injured
tissue for instance, or to rapidly manufacture new ones—for example,
during pregnancy as the uterus increases its volume, so it will need to
speed up the cell cycle.

The stages of the cell cycle are very complex and are regulated
with exquisite accuracy so that, in those cells undergoing division, the
DNA of the mother cell will be correctly transmitted to each of the two
daughter cells. But the regulation cannot be perfect every time and
transcription errors and anomalies inevitably occur from time to time
during the copying process. A detailed knowledge of the mechanisms
involved in normal DNA transfer from cell to cell was crucial to understanding the genesis of cancer at the molecular level and contributed to
the development of medicinal compounds that were capable of acting
at different phases of the cycle of cell division. These very active compounds operate at highly specific locations of the cycle, but they induce
very general and widespread unwanted effects elsewhere in the body,
and furthermore their effectiveness diminishes over time, as other cells
in the body dampen and resist their action.

Development of cancer: a long story

Cancer is the outcome of a slow process of disequilibrium over many
years. Long before tumors become detectable, disturbances have been
in place in the individual's body. There are several phases.

The *preclinical* or *phase of initiation* is the first step, and derives from
an abnormality in the genome of a single cell that will gradually reduce
its ability to operate normally and will eventually transform it into a
cancerous cell.

This cancerous cell may be destroyed by the defense systems of the body, or it may remain in this potentially malignant state until, and the whole body will necessarily be involved, it may progress to the next stage. Under the effect of multiple factors (in which cytokines, growth factors, and angiogenesis will be implicated), this second stage, the *phase of promotion*, will allow the emergence of transformed cellular clones. These will escape the overall control of the immune systems. By the time a tumor becomes detectable, the cancer has entered the *clinical phase*. This is characterized by the risk of cancerous cells invading neighboring tissues, and spreading either the through bloodstream or the lymphatic system. This is what is meant by the development of metastatic cancer.

Finally, if no treatments are able to stop these phenomena, the disease enters its *terminal phase*.

Detection is not prevention

By the time the tumor is detectable by scans, ultrasound and other such techniques, it is already rather late in the process. The length of time between the development of the first abnormal cell and the stage at which the tumor becomes detectable is estimated to be between 5 and 7 years. To reach this clinically noticeable stage, the single rogue cell will have undergone approximately 30 cell doublings, giving rise to a tumor of approximately 10^9 cells, weighing about 1 g. The average growth and development of tumors is summarized in the following table:

Phase	Notes
1 Preclinical	Clinically undetectable
	Typically, 3–4 times longer than the clinical phase
	Can last 8 years (in breast cancer, for example)
2 Clinical	Threshold for detection of the disease reached
	1 g of tumor = 10^9 cells = 30 cellular doublings from the initial cell
3 Terminal	1 kilo of tumor = 10^{12} cells = additional ten doublings

Great progress in early detection has been made by the powerful imaging techniques available to modern medicine, but as the table above illustrates, once you discover that your tumor is malignant it is already too late to prevent it. Is there not another more *timely* way, to monitor our patients so that when we observe metabolic and hormonal tendencies that might predispose towards the development of cancer, we can intervene at an early stage?

The point at which cancer becomes irreversible is in the order of 1 million malignant cells but the point at which it becomes *detectable* is 1 billion cancer cells, a thousand times larger. Treatment of the tumor at this late stage, by whatever means, can hardly deserve to be described as cancer prevention. Detection is not prevention.

True prevention has to be initiated long before cancer manifests. It involves searching for and correcting all the elements that, over the years, permitted the initial abnormal cell, little by little, to develop undetected, before the cancer finally came to light. We urgently need a comprehensive approach, one that places the individual person at the center of our treatment and management of the disease. This approach explains how malfunctions in the endocrine system allowed this kind of disease to take hold.

Programed death of cells: apoptosis

Cells are living functional units that follow a very precise life cycle that determines their development, renewal, and their death. Every day, 200,000 million cells die while others are born. They are programmed to perform specific functions for a defined length of time. If a cell fails to be recognized by its neighbors, a self-destruct mechanism is triggered, whereby the cell is eliminated. a constantly operating genetic program underpins this cell death, which is known as apoptosis.

This cell destruction appears to be an instrument of death, but in reality, it is a mechanism that ensures life: destruction in the service of construction. Apoptosis is also involved in the immune response and in cellular repair. In the event of a bacterial infection, our white cells flood the circulation to detect and eliminate them. After they have mounted resistance against the infection, the nucleus of the cells involved gives the order to self-destruct, and so they disappear, as if by magic.

As constant a phenomenon as cell division itself, apoptosis orchestrates the destruction of cells once they lose their ability to divide. At each cell division, the chromosomes lose some of their telomeres. These are regions of non-coding sequences at each end of a chromosome, and are thought to protect it from deterioration while it uncoils during the duplication of the cell, rather like a cap on a thread to prevent it fraying.

Also, telomeres may prevent the incorrect fusion of neighboring chromosomes; it is theorized that their gradual shortening is integral to the aging process. After a number of cell divisions, as telomeres shorten and cellular functions deteriorate such cells are given the signal to end their lives. Stem cells are somewhat exempt from this process on account of the enzyme telomerase they generate to prevent premature aging and death. Some cancers also possess this enzyme and so are able to resist apoptosis.

Another protection against unregulated cell division involves so-called anti-oncogenes. These genes protect the integrity of DNA against damage from, for example, the threat of an overwhelming viral infection, and also mitigate the negative effects of certain genetic abnormalities. They do so by coding for special proteins that inhibit mitosis.

If the DNA can be repaired by the maintenance systems within the cell nucleus, the cycle resumes. But if repair cannot be achieved, the nucleus of the abnormal cells orders its own destruction by apoptosis. This mechanism of apoptosis is especially important during the virus attacks, because without it, the damaged cells would die by necrosis, which is a messy and destructive pathway, and leaves the tissue vulnerable to diseases such as multiple sclerosis or cancer.

Apoptosis also occurs as a natural physiological phenomenon, for example, during a woman's menstrual cycle. In the early phase of the cycle, the lining of the womb thickens under the influence of estrogens. This proliferation of cells is necessary to provide a suitable bed into which a fertilized ovum may implant itself. If fertilization does not occur, the levels of estrogen drop and the thickened lining is programmed to self-destruct, partly by apoptosis. This results in menstruation, when the cycle begins again. When control of this natural cycle of rapid cell multiplication (or hyperplasia) is lost, a woman is prone to develop adenomas and fibroids. If this situation coexists with viral infections, or if endocrine disruptors are present at the same time, there is a greater likelihood of a turn toward dysplasia and, sooner or later, this may cause a carcinoma to develop in the wall of the womb or in the cervix.

From normal to cancerous cell

A person's individual genetic makeup plays an important role in the transformation of a normal cell into a cancerous cell. Some genes may trigger this transformation when they are activated, while others, conversely, do it when they are switched off, indicating that they may exert some protective function. Extensive genetic research has tried to identify both pathological and protective genes and to work out to what extent they are involved in the development of cancer. We will look at how far these research efforts take us and, with their limitations the hopes, but also the fears they generate.

A fundamental point to grasp is that a gene can only be expressed or inactivated in response to a metabolic demand from our body. This concept is crucial to ridding ourselves of a misconception about our genome: the idea that everything is programmed from our origin by an absolute determinism so that our fate is sealed and the outcome inevitable is just plain wrong. Only by considering the body as a whole in its entirety (physical, emotional, and spiritual), can we understand why a particular gene is turned on or off. We need to understand its relationship with its environment, whatever that might be, to know whether the outcome is likely to be pathological. Certainly, our genes determine many aspects of ourselves, but we are infinitely more than our genes! Aspects of our behavior can be modified over time and their intensity and expression altered. Inappropriate behaviors, out of character and contrary to our interests, play an adverse role in our health especially when we ignore their effects or are in denial about them. We can turn away from the inevitable. We have a large number of strategies we can put to good use to change the course of our health and our destiny.

Faced with a research industry dedicated almost exclusively to the search for "the" miracle molecule that will make cancer "disappear," we need to take our health into our own hands. Fortunately, there has been a growth in recent years of lifestyle measures and medical trends which emphasize the role each one of us can play in reducing the current rise in cancer and the deterioration in public health, which is reflected in the huge increase in the cost of healthcare.

Aggressions

Our way of life is characterized by disturbance on so many levels! Starting with the pollution that affects us all, obvious or hidden: fruit and vegetables contaminated with pesticides, fish with mercury, meat loaded with antibiotics and hormones, water contaminated by industrial effluent, genetically modified cereals, lifeless foods colored with artificial dyes, air pollutants dispersed in the air we breathe, noise pollution, the frantic pace of work, the burdens of professional life, with competition ruling all of our lives. The sources of our imbalances are manifold.

Each one of these aggressors on their own might seem rather harmless but when all of them are added together, the impact can overwhelm our body's recuperative powers, as are the frenetic stresses we impose upon it, failing to respect the day/night cycle. This disturbs the settings in our biological clocks and prevents our sleep from being fully restorative.

Our overtaxed bodies may then also suffer the onslaught inflicted by modern medicine, which has rather got carried away in the race to provide potent synthetic medicines for generalized use, the effects of which are beyond immediate control. Children are stuffed with antibiotics immediately after birth, pricked on all sides by a series of upsetting vaccines, the obese are prescribed treatments like Mediator®, the elderly are overloaded with anti-inflammatory drugs for their rheumatic ailments, the depressed are knocked out by sleeping pills, or agitated by antidepressants, the menopausal women are dosed up with hormones. So many products thoughtlessly prescribed where in many cases a little common sense would have gone a long way. Other measures would have made such powerful drugs unnecessary, such as the initiation of good habits of physical and mental hygiene from a very early age, and the use of less aggressive therapies, so much more appropriate to our physiology.

When cancer becomes generalized

The unrelenting and varied nature of these aggressors will inevitably upset the equilibrium of our body, and so will disrupt the normal operation of our genes and is more likely to light the fuse of destructive ones.

Modern life, which questions the value of self-discipline, makes healthy living quite difficult. These trends create and promote imbalances, against which the body has to constantly respond. Until one day, when unable to continue the struggle, some cells manage to acquire their own autonomy. They thus escape from central control and generate disordered, anarchic tissue. This is cancer. The path to cancer, whether short or long, is specific and characteristic to each individual.

It is the condition in which cells turn their back on community life and parasitize neighboring normal cells. In order to grow and multiply, they force the nearby cells to provide them with nourishment, which progressively leads to the destruction of the surrounding healthy tissue.

They ensure their growth and survival by diverting the systems of the body and capturing nutrients for their own benefit. They disrupt the normal functioning of the endocrine system, which is then no longer able to ensure the coherent management of the entire body. They subvert that the production of growth factors which enables them to grow apace, to the detriment of the body on which they feed. As their number grows, they will take a larger and larger share of the energy they have diverted from healthy tissues. Eventually they become discernible as a small tumor.

Then, by a process known as angiogenesis, the tumor attracts new lymph and blood vessels to itself in order to provide the oxygen and nutrients needed by all growing tissue. Small tumors cluster together and attract the white cells normally responsible for defense. These leucocytes are subverted into stimulating the inflammatory response so that instead of destroying them, they will go on to do the opposite and generate even more abnormal cell activity and facilitates their spread throughout the body.

As they pass freely through the bloodstream and lymphatic vessels, they have to confront circulating cells of the immune system and those that act as filters to protect the liver and lungs. As they circulate, they stimulate platelets in the blood to create tiny clots, which they use as camouflage. Protected by these micro-clots, they synthesize enzymes that will enable them to invade and attach to new tissue and proliferate.

A crucial stage of the disease has now been reached with the emergence of metastases in the lymph nodes and in other organs distant from the site of the original tumor. Their aggressiveness does not end there. They are able to survive in very difficult conditions and defy normal cell death by synthesizing telomerase (or telomere terminal transferase), the same enzyme made by stem cells. By reconstituting the telomeres of the chromosomes, they prevent apoptosis and so the cancer cells are able to divide uncontrollably. Their aggressive power becomes limitless and so control over life seeps away from the sufferer.

Research into powerful treatments

Faced with the damage caused by these abnormal cells, it was a logical therapeutic aim to find ways and means to fight back against them. The pharmaceutical industry strove to develop very particular weapons that targeted those cellular micro-mechanisms that had been derailed, aiming at destroying the anarchic cells as they developed. Alkylating agents, antimetabolites, vegetable alkaloids, topoisomerase inhibitors, antitumor antibiotics, and others were tried, and thus chemotherapy was born. The clear objective—to destroy cancer cells—seems to have been attained. Chemotherapy agents produce dramatic results very quickly, but they are so toxic that they cause many grievous side effects, mostly consequent on the damage they cause to healthy cells.

Unfortunately, the early promise of these products has been short lived, and the initial high hopes have been dashed. In a large number of cases, the cancerous cells seem to have been eradicated, only to reappear, after a long or short interval, and when they do so they become even more aggressive because, having survived the action of the anticancer drug, they have become resistant to it.

The race is on to find other more potent molecules, which would attack every part of the cell, apart from the genes themselves, supplemented by other means such as hormones therapy, or immunotherapy with cytokines. This has given rise to many more active products; while these are effective, they are also very toxic. They have scarcely been used as their limitations soon became evident: cancer cells speedily bypass their action and the survival rates have been much shorter than expected and hoped for.

A novel strategy aims to block cancer's ability to induce the formation of new blood vessels, thereby reducing their ability to obtain nutrients. These anti-angiogenesis drugs (of which Avastin is the best known) are designed to oppose this single mechanism without fully taking into account how it is connected with and managed by the whole body. But such an analytic approach has its limitations if it is not accompanied by an integrative approach.

There has been a great deal of talk in the press about the great hopes promised by "personalized medicine for cancer" and "targeted therapies" that to hope to destroy cancers by disabling their molecular pathways: tyrosine kinase inhibitors, apoptosis inducers, hormone and immunological therapy. But do these treatments, vaunted as personalized, take into account the individual patient, with all his or her particularities and personalities? No, not at all. These are method-ologies that assess an individual's risk of developing certain cancers according to their genetic makeup and, based on these specific findings, aim to determine how the tumor will react to the molecule in question. Thus, in a case of acute lymphoblastic leukemia that is Philadelphia chromosome-positive (Ph+), the optimal treatment currently proposed combining chemotherapy with a BCR-ABL tyrosine kinase inhibitor, Imatinib (Glivec®).[12] But where is the individual patient in all of this?

To give another example, women suffering from HER2-positive[13] breast cancer run a greater risk of rapid growth and dissemination of their tumor, compared to those with breast cancers that are HER2-negative. For them, a targeted treatment using trastuzumab (Herceptin®) to block specific molecules that promote the growth of cancer, will be more effective than conventional therapy. In both cases, the equation is as follows: gene identified ⇒ particular tumor present ⇒ treatment tar-geting the tumor. But where does the patient in his or her totality enter into this equation?

Knowing that one chemical substance is more effective than another on a cancer cell is certainly progress. But, it still applies the same simpli-fying methodology which always looks at "the disease" at the molecular level: applies standardized protocols according to "the type of tumor," prescribes identical repetitive treatment to all patients with "the same" genetic abnormality and with "the same" tumor. But where does the ill person figure in all of this? If only the oncologist would take the indi-vidual patient into account when formulating the therapeutic strategy, we might hope for a better outcome from these targeted treatments.

Cancer: the concept of terrain is of paramount importance

Cancer cannot be disconnected from the individual. You don't get cancer by bad luck! It is not a matter of chance: it sneaks in, and is many years in the making. It results from a set of physiological imbalances that silently progress and eventually cause a cell, or a group of cells, to escape from the overall control of the body. Without our being aware of it, we have an alert system that protects us from the risk of dangerous cells being created and transformed into a tumor. This silent system operates surreptitiously, day by day.

If this system of natural protection gradually loses its effectiveness, after a variable period of time, a tumor will make itself known. Cancer is part of the body that generated it, and is deep-rooted and feeds on it and develops to its detriment. All aspects of the patient's body is implicated in the establishment and development of a cancer long before it makes an appearance, during the treatment and even afterwards. This justifies the need for the permanent monitoring of every patient and a treatment formulated that would be appropriate to his or her terrain.

Aggressors in oncology

The body's inability to deal with the development of abnormal cells is proportionate to the intensity and length of time it has been exposed to carcinogens. But the role of these, however important they might appear, is not as fundamental as we have been led to believe. A new approach is needed to understand that each individual responds differently to aggressors by the according to the specific structure of his or her terrain. We are not denying the role of the aggressor, but is it not legitimate to examine it in the context of the unique individual it attacks?

Let us take the example of smoking. It is regarded as the main cause of lung cancer. However, there are people who have smoked 20 cigarettes a day for 30 years and who are in perfect shape and others who do not smoke and yet develop this type of cancer. This leads us to consider that if smoking is the main factor, it is not sufficient in itself to trigger the disease and the specific structure of the individual must also play a fundamental role.

Consider the important increase in the incidence of lung cancer in women in the last 10 years: it is estimated that it will equal the incidence of breast cancer by 2025. Certainly, the fact that more and more women smoke plays an undeniable role in this increase, but tobacco alone does not seem sufficient to explain it. Indeed, recent studies are beginning to point to the role played by estrogens in the rise of this type of cancer, making them more susceptible than men to the deleterious effects of tobacco. A study published in 2011[14] found that estrogens increase the risk of developing cancer in the head or neck in young women. Another study has shown that cigarette smoke increases the activity of estrogens in the lungs of mice which correlated with the number of lung cancers they went on to develop.

There is clearly a link between the aggressor, which is tobacco, the terrain, an excess of estrogen, and lung cancer. This demonstrates an indivisible triptych: the aggressor, the affected person, and the disease.

The current approach to cancer, by contrast, takes into account only the aggressor (tobacco) and the disease (lung cancer).

The clinical research we are engaged in encourages us to go further still and adopt an even more comprehensive approach: one that is not limited to considering only the role of estrogens, but how the body needs be studied in its entirety to give us a better understanding of the risks woman run when faced with a carcinogen. Then, armed with detailed knowledge of the entire internal state, we will be in a better position to provide a truly preventative treatment. This line of thinking is valid for all types of aggressors confronting any individual in their lifetime, particularly when these aggressors are lurking in our environment, such as the endocrine disruptors discussed in Chapter 8.

People may rightly be worried about the risks they run by consuming food containing additives and sweeteners, which are known carcinogens. However, the outcome will not be the same for two people living under the same roof and eating the same processed foods for decades: the changes that these products will induce and the risk of developing cancer will depend upon the terrain of each individual. A comparable situation is found with prolonged exposure to chemical pollutants, deemed to be carcinogenic. Two farmers working in neighboring fields who annually spray their crops with the same pesticides will not necessarily develop the "same" diseases. One will develop a devastating cancer of the pancreas 20 years later, while the other will be perfectly happy and continue to cultivate his grains. This illustrates the importance of the state of each individual's terrain.

Of course, the longer one is exposed to a potentially carcinogenic substance, the greater the likelihood of developing cancer. In extreme cases, when a person suffers massive poisoning, all the defenses of the body are overwhelmed and its ability to regulate itself is destroyed. This happened to people contaminated by toxic doses of radioactive fallout following the Chernobyl disaster. Sooner or later this triggered serious side effects in most of them, some of them dying from leukemia.

Cancer screening tests

The marketing of genetic testing for cancer risk has really taken off and is expected to double, reaching $5 billion in 2012. Mutations in the genes are the principle source of an inherited predisposition to cancer. These mutations belong to three major groups: tumor suppressor genes, genes that assure the general stability of the genome, and onco-genes. Many genes may be involved in the onset of a whole range of pathologies, such as colon polyps, stomach cancer, retinoblastoma, kidney cancers, skin cancers, or brain tumors. But the results provided by these tests pose problems of interpretation: a negative test does not mean that the cancer will not occur; conversely, they may also throw up false positives.

The situation is made even more complex by many other factors, related to the baseline physiological state but also to the individual's diet and emotional state that will influence the expression of a known risk. There is a great deal of difference between a potential risk and one that is expressed. Not everyone carrying the gene for a disease will develop that disease. Modern science has yet to quantify the rela-tionship between the genetic abnormality and the expression of frank disease. In our view, these relationships may be explained only by con-sidering and understanding the role that the individual plays in trigger-ing the expression of the pathogenic gene. It means, in other words, that the state of an individual's organs, functions and dynamic regulation should be considered in all their totality.

Let us take the example of a woman whose mother, grandmother, and sister have all developed breast cancer. Because of the high familial predisposition to this disease, family members can undergo genetic screening to detect if they are carriers of BRCA1 or BRCA2 gene muta-tions. These are known to pose a very high risk of early-onset aggres-sive cancers of breast and ovaries. Even if the test proves negative, the woman cannot be sure that she will not develop cancer any more than a woman who does not carry the abnormal gene. If the test is positive, what are the options for her doctor?

That this woman runs a high risk of developing a cancer is certain. But the geneticist cannot know when, or how, or why this risk will materialize, only that a time bomb lies deep within her body. What advise can the doctor give his patient? To monitor it, of course: closer clinical scrutiny, mammograms, ultrasounds, and so on. But are these checks really going to help? The chances are that the benefits of this type of "monitoring" are limited to discovering that the risk has been transformed into a real cancer!

Even though her physician knows that his patient is carrying this dangerous gene there are no really effective therapeutic measures that can change the course of things. In very high-risk cases the course proposed is the surgical removal of both breasts. Prophylactic bilateral mastectomy is said to "constitute a very efficient protection against the risk of breast cancer [sic]"; surgery sometimes includes the removal of both ovaries.[15]

The equation is as follows: dangerous gene present ⇒ risk of occurrence of a serious tumor ⇒ no preventative medical treatment ⇒ preventative removal of both breasts. But where is the human being in all of this?

Improving the quality of screening

Couldn't we find less radical solutions? If a woman develops the disease one day, it is because "something," at a certain time in her life, has changed in her entire body. And this "something," which is a change in the overall equilibrium of her terrain, will trigger cancer after a shorter or longer period of gestation. Why does modern medicine not study the changing physiological mechanisms in this woman's body that over time will cause the genetic gun to go off?

Even if biological markers are developed that can accurately predict the outcome of these cancers, we should take the advice of Professor Olivier Cussenot:[16] "we must remember the simple things. Currently, a family history of early cancer is a more important factor in assessing the risks than genetic markers in human blood."

The Endobiogenic approach to individuals suffering from cancer studies the links between the cancer and the totality of the patient. It allows a better understanding of all the associated abnormalities that contribute to the onset of the disease. As chance has no place in physiology, the adverse power of the abnormal gene can only be triggered because the body sanctions it.

By allowing us to quantify the evolution of the biological mechanisms that underpin the disease, the Biology of Functions is a vital tool for identifying the trends towards cancer in an individual so that we can put real preventative measures in place. it could, for example, help identify the reasons why a pathological gene induced cancer in a 30-year-old woman but not in her 60-year-old mother, even though she carries the same gene.

The prevailing medical attitude causes huge distress: "you have the gene but there is nothing we can do except monitor it and wait and see; we will do our best to detect the disease the moment it appears and then we will remove your breast." We could instead adopt a positive attitude and offer preventative measures.

Once we have identified the imbalances in the patient's terrain, we can help maintain it in equilibrium by prescribing treatments to correct these imbalances. Preliminary studies that we have conducted in this area lead us to formulate the hypothesis that abnormalities in at least three hormonal axes favors the triggering of these pathological genes. Namely, that an excess of estrogens with abnormal activity of the thyroid axis is coupled with excessive anabolism of the somatotropic axis, in which human growth hormone stimulates construction in the body. Other specific imbalances also have a part to play.

It would not be difficult to organize a preliminary short and inexpensive study, fulfilling all the criteria of modern science, to test the basic soundness of such a hypothesis. One of the obstacles to be overcome is to convince analytical sciences of the positive results that a synthetic approach to biology could contribute to the understanding of disease. The great problem that confronts genetics is the interpretation of the results of genetic tests. This arises precisely from an absence of an integrative approach to the data obtained.

So far, modern medicine has singularly failed to explore the notion that every cancer is specific and particular to the individual who develops it. Understanding the specific physiological links between an individual and his or her cancer would give the oncologist insights into why the onset, rapidity of growth and developmental features of one patient's cancer are different from those of another, even though their cancers are similar.

Offering patients better outcomes: complementarity between endobiogeny and heavy treatments

A very precise clinical examination is a precondition for diagnosing the terrain of an ill person. The doctor should not focus attention solely on the part of the body in which the cancer is found, but should make every effort to identify the subtlest sign anywhere in the body that (either by its presence or its absence) may lead to an understanding of the physiological functioning of the patient. This will provide the clinician with important clues linking the tumor with the person and to better assess how the disease has developed and the likely response to treatment.

The Biology of Functions, by giving such a clear overview of the functioning of the entire body, provides quantitative data that indicate which biological systems are failing and permits the development of the patient's condition to be followed in a quantifiable manner. Equipped with this data from the outset, the doctor is able to make a more accurate assessment of the situation and so will act as a more precise guide to the optimal treatments: surgery, radiotherapy, or chemotherapy, as appropriate. The side effects caused by heavyweight chemotherapy especially in the digestive system, on the liver and on the immune system involving the destruction of white blood cells should be counterbalanced by an appropriate parallel treatment. The environmental factors most likely to aggravate the disease should also be considered from the onset.

Diet is such an important factor in the management of cancer and needs to be tailored to the individual patient and support the liver in its work of decontamination of the cell detritus created by the chemotherapy. At the same time, the treatment needs to correct the root causes of the disease and to limit the risk of proliferation of the cancer. It needs to reposition the state of the terrain and shift it towards a new Endobiogenic equilibrium, helping the patient establish peaceful coexistence with his or her cancer, now under control, and also to minimize the likelihood of the cancer being reactivated in the future.

At the end of the consultation, the doctor must take the time to explain to the patient the dysfunctions that have brought about the illness and led to its progression so that the necessity of the prescribed treatment can be fully appreciated. Fortified with a clear understanding of the way in which his or her body works, its strengths and its weaknesses, the patient can embrace and own a real change of lifestyle, a new way of being to minimize the damage done to his or her body. The part played by the patient is essential to healing. The more clearly the patient understands the need to take into their own hands the management of their disease, the greater the chances of success. A commitment to the prescribed therapeutic in close collaboration with his or her doctor can only improve the effectiveness of the treatment, independently of any placebo effect. Changes in lifestyle will bring about significant physiological benefits. a personalized diet will play an important part, as will techniques that reduce the negative effects of stress: psychotherapy, meditation, relaxation, yoga and the like.

New perspectives?

It is very difficult to arouse interest in new ways of thinking and to bring innovation into the conservative field of oncology even if promising results of scientific work, carried out with all due rigor, ought to attract oncologists' attention. If a publication tries to question any of the certainties and tenets of current mainstream belief, it is nigh impossible to establish genuine debate and to promote new knowledge and to allow a synthesis between orthodox medicine and other treatment options.

Dr. Simon Schraub, Director of the Center for Fight Against Cancer of Strasbourg, cancer specialist, reported[17] a few years ago the results of several studies conducted in China on patients with various cancers. Each year, more than a million cancer patients are treated in that country by conventional methods: surgery, radiotherapy, chemotherapy, or hormone therapy. In order to increase the effectiveness of these standard methods, they often combine them with medicinal plants as complementary or symptomatic treatments. The researchers Cheng and Liu, in a randomized study of 52 patients, showed that *Lycium barbarum* increased the efficiency of radiotherapy in uncomplicated carcinoma of the lung. The treated group had a rate of overall remission (complete and partial response) of 92%, while for the control group the rate was 58%. in another randomized study on 100 cases, Zhang demonstrated that both *Ilex asprella* and *Ilex pubescens* are able to augment the effectiveness of radiotherapy in nasopharyngeal carcinoma. After three months of treatment, 100% of the group receiving both radiotherapy and Phytotherapy went into complete remission, while only 71% of the group receiving radiotherapy alone attained remission.

According to the Chinese doctors who conducted these and other equally promising studies, the positive results observed are best explained by improved immune functions, protection of the bone marrow, which produces blood cells, regulation of the endocrine and enzymatic activity in the body, better removal of waste; these benefits also meant there were fewer complications from the treatment and a reduction in the spread of tumors. It has to be said that other Chinese research, which use this kind of approach even more extensively, are much less promising. There is no evidence that medicinal plants used in these studies were able to cure cancer in patients with advanced stages of disease any more than chemotherapy could. Yet, overall, these studies show that patients treated by protocols that included medicinal plants had very favorable median survival times, but these results have never been well received in our country. Is that the result of simple prejudice against any protocol that includes medicinal plants?

We should heed the advice of the great French physiologist, Claude Bernard when he wrote, "if an idea is presented to us, we should not reject it just because it fails to agree with the expected outcomes predicted by established theory."[18] These studies have been overlooked not because the results presented by these physicians were questionable but because it is the practice to reject new ideas without even trying to analyze the results, under the cloak of unfounded claims that the "clinical studies seem questionable with respect to methodology and evaluation of the results" without providing any evidence for such statements. Perhaps we should listen to the words of Henri Poincaré, another great Frenchman, when he said: *to doubt everything and to believe everything are two equally convenient solutions; both dispense with the necessity of reflection.*[19]

How can modern medicine reject out of hand the very idea that medicinal plants could provide positive outcomes for cancer patients, when it has never incorporated them into conventional treatment protocols? Even skeptical scientists should not reject new findings before even considering them? Shouldn't such findings be tested by a series of low-cost studies conducted in French hospitals, given the potential benefits for cancer patients? Such studies would aim to corroborate the validity of the reports or, on the contrary, to invalidate them. It is a pity that such research has not been funded, as the fight against cancer has proved very difficult, and is one in which pharmaceutical companies can spend $4–$5 billion to test a patentable molecule that might give patients an extra four or five months of life.

Now that we have reached the end of this final chapter, what conclusion can we come to? Medicine has more and more success in treating patients with cancer and in reducing deaths from the disease, but a cure is still not in sight. It has powerful weapons for intervening, often preventing a flare-up, either by the surgical removal of the tumor, or by attacking it with radiotherapy or chemotherapy in cases where it poses a risk of spreading. New methods that target the physiological mechanisms at work in the tumor more accurately represent an important step forward in terms of efficacy. Finally, medicinal products developed to combat some of the adverse effects of chemotherapy, such as nausea and vomiting and drop in white blood cells, will undeniably improve the outcomes and patient comfort.

These represent considerable advances in the management of the disease, yet modern medicine has not been successful in developing preventative strategies to halt the dramatic rise in the number of new cases. In prevention, it has considered only known aggressors such as tobacco and other harmful lifestyles, but these represent only partially the many factors involved in the initiation of cancer, and falls short of true prevention, which involves a full understanding of the individual person.

Nor have the advances in genetics and the search for genes involved in the expression of cancers, led to the development of truly preventative methods. It has not been able to prevent recurrence of the disease nor predict who will fail to respond to treatment. The extension of life expectancy that new molecules and protocols have achieved has been modest: a few months at most. The high cost of such treatments puts their widespread use out of the reach of the public healthcare system, which raises difficult ethical questions.

Why not, then, take advantage of this new approach to the treatment of patients who suffer from cancer?

CONCLUSION

Modern medicine is confronted with a difficult paradox. The funding devoted to research has never been so great, and medical technology has never made such progress as in the last two decades.

- With new techniques of resuscitation, it is now possible to revive people who previously would have been beyond all hope.
- Developments in surgery mean that failing organs can safely be replaced.
- Sophisticated devices allow deep structures of the human body to be visualized in minutest detail.
- Fundamental research in genetics has unraveled the secrets of the human body.
- State-of-the-art pharmaceutical research has produced medicinal products that can alter the course of serious disease.

However, never before has medicine been confronted with a crisis on such a scale, and the healthcare system is close to breaking point.

- Too many scandals have surfaced. Scandals related to medicinal products, conflicts of interest, products deemed safe enough that soon prove dangerous and have to be taken off the market a few years later.
- There is an urgent need to make access to quality care available to everyone, to bring some hope of true health.

Despite the huge sums of money being spent, the research endeavor struggles to obtain the results it hopes to find, or to resolve the ethical problems raised. This dilemma bids us to reevaluate the fundamental assumptions on which modern medicine to human life is based.

Even though the methods pioneered by Pasteur have undoubtedly been fruitful, they have now come up against their limits. In fragmenting the human body into its myriad components and separating the part from the whole, rather than envisioning its totality, it has been singularly unable to put the parts back together and to place the human being at the center of the system.

It is perhaps time to bring new ways of thinking into the heart of modern medicine, and create a truly integrated synthesis at all levels of care. Such an approach should start from listening to the patient, examining him or her, analyzing the findings of objective biological tests, establishing a personalized treatment. It needs to be oriented towards research and the development of new medicines and modalities, with prevention being always the dominant aim.

One of the solutions for today's dilemmas and for tomorrow's medicine to flourish will surely embrace an integrative approach, without abandoning the advances made by analytical science. The Endobiogenic approach to medical practice is based on scientific data and on over 40 years of clinical practice, corroborated by many doctors working in France and many other countries. It offers this integrative approach and provides simple and effective methodologies that could be implemented without delay.

For the greater good of those who are sick as well as those in good health, all it would take is for those who have decision-making power in political, scientific, and medical spheres would take immediate and decisive action on a number of measures based on the ideas presented in this book, such as:

- To organize training seminars for physicians under the supervision of the Ministry of Health with the objective of instructing them in the use of medicines with less iatrogenic potential when treating common disorders. Powerful pharmacological medication should be reserved for treatment of last resort;

- To set up healthcare centers in public hospitals, for example, in the Paris Public Hospital System (*Assistance Publique*), similar to those established in Mexico City by the Mexican Ministry of Health;
- To organize both clinical and biological integrative research initiatives in hospitals;
- To use natural-based therapeutic means to support those who are undergoing chemotherapy, and to help support those in palliative care;[1]
- To introduce integrative medicine onto the medical education curriculum;
- To establish patients' associations with the purpose of educating patients and helping them take responsibility for their own care in a more comprehensive approach to health;
- To encourage the pharmaceutical industry to research, design, and formulate natural-based healthcare products that meet the appropriate scientific criteria; these to be used by the general public as front-line therapy;
- To educational programs on the use of natural-based products in the context of well-ordered self-medication;
- To institute horticultural and agricultural programs for the cultivation of medicinal plants in the immense acreage of fallow land, in tandem with a body responsible for the assurance of the pharmaceutical quality of the crops;
- To create multidisciplinary centers for the Quality Control and evaluation of these proposals;
- To establish international collaborations with countries already involved in these new lines of research such as the United States, Belgium, Great Britain, Mexico, and Tunisia and to extend the education and research effort to other interested countries.

This message is addressed to all those having decision-making power. Our future and that of our children depends upon their positive response.

APPENDIX ONE

Endocrine disruptors, a danger for every one of us

A few examples, from a long list

There follows a quick overview of products that present a real threat to our health and that of our children.

Causing abnormalities and malformations

Diethylstilbestrol (Distilbene®). This medicine was prescribed in France between 1948 and 1977 to prevent the occurrence of early miscarriage. This product has caused significant genital abnormalities: malformations, sterility, and cancer in tens of thousands of children born to women for whom it was prescribed. The damage extends to their grandchildren, and so has involved three generations.[1]

Causing sterility

The *parabens* constitute a ubiquitous group of preservatives found in cosmetics, creams, lotions, shampoos, gels, cleaners, lipstick, and toothpaste.[2] They are also used in the food industry (additives E214 to E219) and are found in more than 400 pharmaceutical products in

261

current use, such as antacid medication, medicines for nausea and vomiting, and even antibiotics.

These substances had for a long time been suspected of having adverse effects on fertility and of being implicated in some estrogen-dependent tumors. In September, 2005, the French Food Safety Agency (AFSSA), decided to continue licensing the use of four of the five most commonly used parabens, in spite of the concerns that had been raised about their harmfulness. In May, 2011, the European Commission's Scientific Committee on Consumer Safety (SCCS) drew up a plan to ban isopropyl- and isobutyl-parabens, while accepting a limited use for propyl and butyl parabens, while defining a threshold concentration that could not be exceeded. The decision to maintain propyl-paraben is strange, considering that when used in syrups for children and is likely to produce feminization of young boys. The AFSSA began a pilot study whose results are be released in 2012. In the meantime, we are all left to run the risks.

Molluskicides

Tributyltin (TBT). This substance enters into the composition of paints applied to the hulls of boats and is extremely harmful to marine mollusks. Entire whelk populations in the North Sea have been wiped out because, with the appearance of a penis and spermatic ducts in females, they became unable to reproduce.[3] In France, the Arcachon basin has been particularly affected by the use of paint containing Tributyltin. The European sting winkle, *Ocenebra erinacea*, completely disappeared because of the sterilization induced by these products between 1980 and 1990. These products can persist in marine sediments for up to 10 years.

Causing abnormal thyroid function

The *PBDEs*, found in flame retardant coatings, are present in our furniture, textiles, electronic products, and cars. These substances are found in household dust and so pose a great risk to children playing on the floor who go on to suck their fingers or bite their nails. A high level of these organic pollutants has found in the blood of a large number of people. They can cause abnormalities in the function of thyroid and reproductive hormones, as well as in the nervous system. The European Community has banned the use of some of these compounds, but as the objects that contain them have a long life, exposure to these substances will pursue us for many years.

Turning oysters hermaphrodite

Alkylphenols are found in pesticides and a wide range of industrial products including detergents, cosmetics and cleaning products. They can cause damage to DNA in human lymphocytes. In the laboratory 4-octylphenol has been observed to stimulate growth in breast cancer cells.[4] Nonylphenol, the annual production of which exceeds 600,000 tons, is not readily biodegradable. It enters the food chain through aerosols and also contaminates the ground water where it is known to feminize fish by mimicking the action of estrogen. As a potent endocrine disruptor, it has been shown to render oysters hermaphrodite. It has been found in many products throughout the food chain, in tomatoes, apples, and bread, and was even found in blood in the umbilical cords of half the newborn babies tested in the Netherlands. In 2003, the German Government prohibited Bayer from manufacturing this product.

Causing prostate and other cancers

The *insecticides* and *organochlorine pesticides*, such as DDT, HCB, Chlordane, Aldrin, Toxaphene, Lindane, are derived from the petrochemical industry and first came into use in the 1940s. With resistance to insecticides on the increase, considerable amounts of these products have been spread on crops and sprayed over watercourses. Not readily biodegradable, and persistent in the environment for more than 10 years, they remain as deadly pollutants of soil and water. Although they have been banned for years (Dieldrin in 1994, Chlordane in 1995), they are still a major source of pollution. DDT has been found in Antarctic ice, as well as in poultry, milk, and drinking water. As they are fat soluble, they pass easily through the skin and their effects are cumulative.

It was not until the 1990s that the scale of their harmfulness was realized. In the months following the accidental pollution of Lake Apopka in Florida, a dramatic reduction in the number of alligators who inhabited its waters was observed and of those that survived, the males had a penis so reduced in size that they could no longer reproduce. Although banned, DDT is still sprayed onto the walls of houses to combat mosquitoes in the fight against malaria.

Putting small children at risk

The *PCBs*, or polychlorinated biphenyls, are obtained from benzene, a hydrocarbon derived from petroleum refining. They have been widely used since the 1980s in the manufacture of medicinal products, plastics, and colorants. They are also found in domestic and industrial devices, particularly in electrical transformers. They have been phased out in most of the industrialized countries, but because they are very persistent, they are still found in water and in fish where they have accumulated in fat. Studies have demonstrated a link between exposure of children to PCBs and a number of developmental disorders including learning difficulties and hearing impairment.[5] These products belong to a category of 12 very toxic chemicals called "persistent organic pollutants," because they are resistant to environmental degradation and pollute the entire food chain.

Contaminated child care centers[6]

Phthalates. In March, 2009, the French Environmental Health Association (Association Santé Environement France, or ASEF) conducted a study on the air quality in ten childcare centers. The French Indoor Air Quality Observatory (OQAI) noted with concern the high levels of three undesirable molecules: phthalates, benzene, and formaldehyde. Benzene is found in the atmosphere and in paintings, formaldehyde in chipboard, synthetic foams and paints and the phthalates in plastics and PVC toys.

   These compounds can cause asthma, but also infertility and cancer. The study also found that all the beds tested in which infants slept emitted formaldehyde at values well above the reference toxic range. Formaldehyde is carcinogenic and the source of a number of respiratory disorders. Understandably concerned parents have signed petitions.

Dangerous baby bottles

The recent story of *bisphenol A* shows very clearly how conflicts of interest can obstruct prompt action when it comes to banning harmful products, even when the health of newborn babies is at stake. This compound is used as a lining in food and beverage cans and in plastic bottles, and also to in line baby's bottles. When they are sterilized, heat releases large amounts of bisphenol A into to the baby's milk. It accumulates in body fat.

In June, 2009, the International Society of Endocrinology declared bisphenol[7] to be an endocrine disruptor, potentially a cause of testicular abnormalities in boys, and obesity and early puberty in girls. It may also be involved in breast and prostate cancer, in cardiovascular and thyroid diseases, and in adult obesity. It took a few months for the AFSSA to admit (January 29, 2010) that when heated, *bisphenol A* can contaminate food and may cause adverse endocrine effects but the Agency declared itself unperturbed about the potential for harm, and downplayed the effects seen in experimental animals as "subtle" and would await for the results of further research before acting.

On June 23, 2010, the sale of baby bottles lined with *bisphenol* was banned in France, a move described by the World Health Organization as premature, with the counterclaim that this molecule does not accumulate in the body. A surprising stance, as a few days earlier, a study published in the scientific press reported that men with high blood levels of bisphenol had more than three times the incidence of low sperm count and poor motility.[8] Evidence from other studies shows a correlation between high levels of bisphenol in the urine with a greater risk of cardiovascular disease, diabetes, and reproductive disorders, and with altered liver function.

The ban on the sale of baby bottles lined with bisphenol did not come into force in the European Union until June 1, 2011. Was that the end of the public health scare about this chemical? We doubt it, as the ban does not extend to other containers containing BPA. It is also present in free form in a large number of cash register and credit card receipts. Several INRA research teams found higher residues of BPA in the bodies of cashiers working in shops and supermarkets.[9]

Bisphenol A has been manufactured on a massive scale for several decades and is widely distributed in the environment. Worldwide production, according to industry data, exceeds 3 million tons a year and can be detected in the bodies of the great majority of the population, particularly in children. No doubt the same goes for the thousands of other unnatural chemicals that inhabit our environment. Perhaps within a few years public health agencies will come to see diseases of mysterious origin!

Whether we like it or not, we are all contaminated, since everything ends up in our bodies: pesticides and insecticides of all kinds, dyes, food additives, polluted vegetables, fruit, meat and fish, and pharmaceutical residues in drinking water. No one can know the true price that eventually will have to be paid.

The dirty dozen

The Stockholm Convention was ratified by 150 countries on May 17, 2004, and is dedicated to the elimination or reduction of 12 persistent and highly toxic organic pollutants dubbed "The Dirty Dozen."[10]

One of them is the infamous *dioxin*, which in a disaster at a chemical plant in Seveso in Italy in 1976 contaminated nearly 40,000 people. The quantity of dioxin released in the explosion was the equivalent to nearly half a million lethal doses for humans. The signs and symptoms of acute poisoning, especially of the skin, is well known, but the chronic toxic effects less so. The data points to a wide number of disorders and abnormalities, with harm to the metabolism, reproduction, the central nervous system, and defective immunity.

The threat is still with us, as these compounds are released into the atmosphere by the incomplete combustion of household and hospital waste in poorly controlled waste incinerators. These contaminate the entire planet, and are found everywhere, in the soil, in streams, in dairy products, meat, fish, and crustaceans. In recent years, Europe has faced a number of serious pollution incidents. In 2006, in the Netherlands, dioxin was found in milk and in animal feed. In July, 2007, it was found in guar gum, an additive that is used as a thickener for meat and dairy products, desserts, or deli meats. In 2008, it was found in pork in Ireland, and in milk in Germany. The list of endocrine disruptors is getting longer.[11]

The future of our descendants may be dangerously compromised if science is not put first and foremost in the service of conscience. In the words of François Rabelais: "science without conscience is but the ruin of the soul."

Sources of scientific reviews of medicinal plants

The following bibliography provides an illustration of some of the scientific studies of plants used in the treatment of the patients whose cases have been presented in this book and is but a selection from the large number of fundamental research projects on medicinal plants. It can be accessed at the following address: http://www.ncbi.nlm.nih.gov/pubmed/

1. **Agrimony (*Agrimonia eupatoria*)**
   Lee K. Y., Hwang L., Jeong E. J., Kim S. H., Kim Y. C., Sung S. H., "Effect of neuroprotective flavonoids of Agrimonia eupatoria on glutamate-induced oxidative injury to HT22 hippocampal cells," *Biosci Biotechnol Biochem*, 2010, 74 (8), pp. 1704–1706. Epub 7/08/2010.

2. **Lady's mantle (*Alchemilla vulgaris*)**
   Jonadet M., Meunier M.-T., Villie F., Bastide J.-P., Lamaison J.-L., "Flavonoids extracted from *Ribes nigrum L* and *Alchemilla vulgaris L*: 1. In vitro inhibitory activities on elastase, trypsin and chymotrypsin. 2. Angioprotective activities compared in vivo," *Pharmacol.*, 1986, 17 (1), pp. 21–27.

3. **Hawthorn (*Crataegus oxyacantha*)**
Tadic V. M., Dobric S., Markovic G. M., Dordevic S. M., Arsic I. A., Menkovic N. R., Stevic T. (Institute for Medicinal Plants Research, Belgrade, Serbia), "Anti-inflammatory, gastroprotective, free-radical-scavenging, and antimicrobial activities of hawthorn berries ethanol extract," *J. Agric. Food Chem.*, 2008, 56 (17), pp. 7700–7709. Epub 08/13/2008.

4. **Bergamot (*Citrus aurantium bergamia*)**
Amantea D., Fratto V., Maida S., Rotiroti D., Ragusa S., Nappi G., Bagetta G., Corasaniti MT. (Department of Pharmacobiology and Center of Neuropharmacology of Normal and Pathological Neuronal Plasticity, UCADH, University of Calabria, Cosenza, Italy), "Prevention of glutamate accumulation and upregulation of phospho-akt may account for neuroprotection afforded by bergamot essential oil against brain injury induced by focal cerebral ischemia in rat," *Int. Rev Neurobiol.*, 2009, 85, pp. 389–405.

5. **Cajeput (*Melaleuca leucadendron*)**
Valdés A. F., Martínez J. M., Lizama R. S., Vermeersch M., Cos P., Maes L. (Department of Parasitology, "Pedro Kourí" Institute of Tropical Medicine, Marianao, La Habana, Cuba), "In vitro antimicrobial activity of the Cuban medicinal plants *Simarouba glauca DC*, *Melaleuca leucadendron L* and *Artemisia absinthium L*," *Mem. Inst. Oswaldo Cruz*, 2008, 103 (6), pp. 615–618.

6. **Cinnamon (*Cynamomum zeylanicum*)**
Maedes G. Jr, Henken R. L., Waldrop G. L., Rahman M. M., Gilman S. D., Kamatou G. P., Viljoen A. M., Gibbons S. (Division of Biochemistry and Molecular Biology, Louisiana State University, Baton Rouge, Louisiana, United States), "Constituents of Cinnamon inhibit bacterial Acetyl CoA carboxylase," *Planta Med.*, 2010, 76 (14), pp. 1570–1575.

7. **Blackcurrant (*Ribes nigrum*)**
Garbacki N., Tits M., Angenot L., Damascus J. (Laboratory of Human Physiology, CHU, University of Liege, Sart Tilman, Belgium), "Inhibitory effects of proanthocyanidins from Ribes nigrum leaves on carrageenin acute inflammatory reactions induced in rats," *BMC Pharmacol.*, 2004, 21 (4), p. 25.

8. **Chrysanthellum (*Chrysanthellum americanum*)**
   http://www.ncbi.nlm.nih.gov/pubmed/16164709
   http://www.ncbi.nlm.nih.gov/pubmed/2698952

9. **Eucalyptus (*Eucalyptus globulus*)**
   Mahmoudzadeh-Sagheb H., Heidari Z., Bokaeian M., Moudi. B., "Anti-diabetic effects of Eucalyptus globulus on pancreatic islets: a stereological study," *Folia Morphol* (Warsz), 2010, 69 (2), pp. 112–118.

10. **Chaste tree (*Vitex agnus castus*)**
    Wuttke W., Jarry H., Christoffel V., Spengler B., Seidlová-Wuttke D. (Department of Clinical and Experimental Endocrinology, University of Göttingen, Germany), "Chaste tree (Vitex agnus castus) pharmacology and clinical indications," *Phytomedicine*, 2003, 10 (4), pp. 348–357.

11. **Griffonia (*Griffonia simplicifolia*)**
    Carnevale G., Di Viesti V., Zavatti M., Zanoli P. (Department of Biomedical Sciences, University of Modena and Reggio Emilia, Modena, Italy), "Anxiolytic-like effect of Griffonia simplicifolia Baill. seed extract in rats," *Phytomedicine*, 2011, 18 (10), pp. 848–851. Epub 11/25/2011.

12. **Mistletoe (*Viscum album*)**
    Hong C. E., Lyu S. Y. (Department of Pharmacy, Yeungnam University, Gyeongbuk, Korea), "The antimutagenic effect of mistletoe lectin (*Viscum album* L var. *coloratum agglutinin*)," *Phytother. Res.*, 2011, doi: 10.1002/ptr. 3639.

13. **Lavender (*Lavandula officinalis*)**
    Woelk H., Schläfke S. (Surgery for psychiatry and psychotherapy, Buseck-Beuern, Germany), "A multi-center, double-blind, randomised study of the Lavender oil preparation Silexan in comparison to Lorazepam for generalized anxiety disorder," *Phytomedicine*, 2010, 17 (2), pp. 94–99. Epub 12/3/2009.

14. **Stoneseed (*Lithospermum officinalis*)**
    Auf'mkolk M., Köhrle J., Gumbinger H., Winterhoff H., Hesch R. D., "Antihormonal effects of plant extracts: Iodothyronine deiodinase of rat liver is inhibited by extracts and secondary metabolites of plants," *Horm. Metab. Res.*, 1984, 16 (4), pp. 188–192.

15. **Alfalfa (*Medicago sativa*)**
Bora K. S., Sharma A. L. R. (Institute of Pharmacy, Solan, Himachal Pradesh, India), "Phytochemical and pharmacological potential of Medicago sativa: A review," *Pharm. Biol.*, 2011, 49 (2), pp. 211–220. Epub 10/25/2010.

16. **Gypsywort (*Lycopus europaea*)**
Beer A. M., Wiebelitz K. R., Schmidt-Gayk H. (Department of True Naturopathy, Ruhr-University Bochum, Hattingen, Germany), "*Lycopus europaeus* (Gypsywort): Effects on the thyroidal parameters and symptoms associated with thyroid function," *Phytomedicine*, 2008, 15 (1–2), pp. 16–22.

17. **Walnut (*Juglans regia*)**
Orhan I. E., Suntar I. P., Akkol E. K. (Department of Pharmacognosy, Faculty of Pharmacy, Gazi University, Ankara, Turkey), "In vitro neuroprotective effects of the leaf and fruit extracts of *Juglans regia L* (walnut) through enzymes linked to Alzheimer's disease and anti-oxidant activity," *Int. J. Food. Sci Nutr.*, 2011, 62 (8), pp. 781–786. Epub 5/31/2011.

18. **Passionflower (*Passiflora incarnata*)**
Aslanargun P., Cuvas O., Dikmen B., Aslan E., Yuksel M. U. (Department of Anesthesiology and Intensive Care Medicine, Ankara Training and Research Hospital, Ankara, Turkey), "*Passiflora incarnata Linneaus* as an anxiolytic before spinal anesthesia," *J. Anesth.*, 2011, doi:10.1007/s00540-011-1265-6.

19. **Petitgrain**
Hawrelak J. A., Cattley T., Myers S. P. (School of Health and Human Sciences, Southern Cross University, Lismore, Australia), "Essential oils in the treatment of intestinal dysbiosis: A preliminary in vitro study," *Altern. Med. Rev.*, 2009, 14 (4), pp. 380–384.

20. **Pichi (*Fabiana imbricata*)**
Reyes M., Schmeda-Hirschmann G., Razmilic I., Theoduloz C., Yánez T., Rodríguez J. A. (Natural Products Laboratory, Chemistry Institute of Natural Resources, University of Talca, Talca, Chile),

"Gastroprotective activity of sesquiterpene derivatives from Fabiana imbricata," *Phytother. Res.*, 2005, 19 (12), pp. 1038–1042.

21. **Salad burnet (*Poterium sanguisorba*)**
Yu T., Lee Y. J., Yang H. M., Han S., Kim J. H., Lee Y., Kim C., Han M. H., Kim M. Y., Lee J., Cho J. Y. (College of Biomedical Science, Institute of Bioscience and Biotechnology, Kangwon National University, Chuncheon, Korea), "Inhibitory effect of *Sanguisorba officinalis* ethanol extract on NO and PGEv(2) production is mediated by suppression of NF-B and AP-1 activation signaling cascade," *J. Ethnopharmacol.*, 2011, 134 (1), pp. 11–17. Epub 9/9/2010.

22. **Pine (*Pinus sylvestris*)**
Ka M. H., Choi E. H., Chun H. S., Lee K. G. J. (Department of Food Science and Technology, Dongguk University, Seoul, Korea), "Antioxidative activity of volatile extracts isolated from Angelica tenuissimae roots, peppermint leaves, pine needles, and sweet flag leaves," *Agric. Food Chem.*, 2005, 53 (10), pp. 4124–4129.

23. **Peony (*Paeonia officinalis*)**
http://www.nutritionreview.org/library/peony.root.php
http://www.ncbi.nlm.nih.gov/pmc/articles/PMC2798846/

24. **Plantain (*Plantago major*)**
Ikawati Z., Wahyuono S., Maeyama K. (Department of Pharmacology Ehime University School of Medicine, Shigenobu-cho, Onsen-gun, Japan), "Screening of several Indonesian medicinal plants for their inhibitory effect on histamine release from RBL-2H3 cells," *J. Ethnopharmacol.*, 2001, 75 (2–3), pp. 249–256.

25. **Horsetail (*Equisetum arvense*)**
Cetojevic-Simin D. D., Canadanovic-Brunet J. M., Bogdanovic G. M., Djilas S. M., Cetkovic G. S., Tumbas V. T., Stojiljkovic B. T. (Department of Experimental Oncology, Oncology Institute of Vojvodina, Sremska Kamenica, Serbia), "Antioxidative and antiproliferative activities of different horsetail (*Equisetum arvense L*) extracts," *J. Med. Food*, 2010, 13 (2), pp. 452–459.

26. **Rosemary (***Rosmarinus officinalis***)**
Takaki I., Bersani-Amado L. E., Vendruscolo A., Sartoretto S. M., Diniz S. P., Bersani-Amado C. A., Cuman R. K. (Department of Pharmacy and Pharmacology, State University of Maringá, Maringá, Paraná, Brazil), "Anti-inflammatory and antinociceptive effects of *Rosmarinus officinalis L* essential oil in experimental animal models," *J. Med. Food*, 2008, 11 (4), pp. 741–746.

27. **Blackberry (***Rubus fructicosus***)**
Alonso R., Cadavid I., Calleja J. M. (Department of Pharmacognosy and Pharmacodynamics, University of Santiago de Compostela, Spain), "A preliminary study of hypoglycemic activity of *Rubus fruticosus*," *Planta Med.*, 1980, 40, pp. 102–106.

28. **Sage (***Salvia officinalis***)**
Carrasco F., Schmidt G., Romero A. L., Sartoretto J. L., Caparroz-Assef S. M., Bersani- Amado C. A., Cuman R. K. (Laboratory of Inflammation, Department of Pharmacy and Pharmacology, State University of Maringá, Maringá, Paraná, Brazil), "Immunomodulatory activity of *Zingiber officinale* Roscoe, *Salvia officinalis* L and *Syzygium aromaticum* L essential oils: Evidence for humor and cell-mediated responses," *J. Pharm. Pharmacol.*, 2009, 61 (7), pp. 961–967.

29. **Thyme (***Thymus vulgaris***)**
Tohidpour A., Sattari M., Omidbaigi R., Yadegar A., Nazemi J. (Department of Bacteriology, School of Medical Sciences, Tarbiat Modares University, Téhéran, Iran), "Antibacterial effect of essential oils from two medicinal plants against Methicillin-resistant *Staphylococcus aureus* (MRSA)," *Phytomedicine*, 2010, 17 (2), pp. 142–145. Epub 7/02/2009.

30. **Linden (***Tilia tomentosa***)**
Viola H., Wolfman C., Levi de Stein M., Wasowski C., Pen~ a C., Medina J. H., Paladini C. (Institute of Cell Biology, Faculty of Medicine Paraguay, Buenos Aires, Argentina), "Isolation of pharmacologically active benzodiazepine receptor ligands from *Tilia tomentosa* (*Tiliaceae*)," *J. Ethnopharmacol.*, 1994, 44 (1), pp. 47–53.

Websites

For patients
  www.phyto2000.org
  www.simepi.info
  http://www.endobiogeny.com/

For physicians
France: www.simepi.info
Mexico: http://sites.google.com/site/someficac/Home
Great Britain: http://brems.org.uk
United States: http://www.endobiogeny.com
              http://www.eimcenter.com

ACKNOWLEDGMENTS

Jean-Claude Lapraz

I dedicate this book: to my patients without whom this book would not exist, for it was they who enriched and taught me true knowledge, that of life; to my wife Nelly and to my children Jean-François, Anne-Marie, Fabienne, Leslie, and Myriam, as well as to Françoise, who knows the length of the road traveled and understands the cost; to Marie-Laure de Clermont-Tonnerre, for having the idea for this book in the first place and had the resolution to see it through to completion, collaborating with me for 2 years, and putting these new concepts into an accessible form for a non-medical public.

This book would not be what it is without the support of my friend Patrice Pauly, with whom I have worked closely for over 10 years and whose opinions are always valuable; we have developed theoretical models and practical research projects together for the promotion of Endobiogeny and the Biology of Functions in the United States and other countries; I thank my friend Christophe Jacquemin, not only for reading the manuscript but also for his wise advice and steadfast support during the final drafts; and also my colleagues and friends, Alain Carillon and Jean-Christophe Charrié, who, despite their heavy workloads, took the time to read it at every stage of the process and gave sound advice, as well as to my friends Gilbert Julliard, Claude Gassmann, Jean-Marc Leblon, Brigitte Rolard, and Louis Charles Oudin for their constant support.

Special mention must be made of Doctors Alain Carillon, Jean-Christophe Charrié, Brigitte Godard, Kamyar Hedayat, Patrice Pauly, Christophe Jacquemin, Guillaume Prache, Josiane Geffroy, Nadine Chauvet, and Claude Gassman, who are co-founders with me of the International Society of Endobiogenic Medicine and Integrative Physiology (SIMEPI). Without them, the development of Endobiogenic Medicine and Clinical Phytotherapy could not have taken place.

Nor should I forget my many colleagues in other countries who, for more than 20 years, have faithfully supported our efforts to promote Endobiogeny in England, in the United States, Mexico, Tunisia, and more recently in China and who participated with us in the creation of the International Federation of Endobiogenic Medicine and Integrative Physiology (FIMEPI). I have to especially thank my friend Kamyar Hedayat, President of the American Society of Endobiogenic Medicine and Integrative Physiology (ASEMIP) for taking overall responsibility for the teaching in the United States; and to my American friends who supported the development of Endobiogeny in their country: Anne-Marie Buhler, Pierre Buhler, Nica George, Ron George, as well as to Doctors Jean Bokelmann, Laramie Wheeler, and Annette Davis CN, and Eric Davis for setting up a teaching program in English along with Dan Kenner, TuVi Luong, and Ruby Shih; to my friend Colin Nicholls in London, President of the British Society for Endobiogenic Medicine; and, in Mexico, to Dr. Paul Hersch tireless traveling companion; he and I, together with Doctors Miguel Poujol, Ana Cecilias Sanchez, and Angela Silva developed a project over 20 years which led to the integration of Clinical Phytotherapy and Endobiogeny into the healthcare system of Mexico City; thanks also to the many others who practice Endobiogeny in healthcare centers in that city; and to Professor Rachid Chemli, who has labored for over 20 years to promote the use of medicinal plants in the Tunisian health care system and to all the members of the Tunisian Society of Clinical Phytotherapy; and in China, to Dr. Steve Xue and to Mrs. Louisa Chan.

Marie-laure de clermont-tonnerre:

I dedicate this book to Jean-François, my husband, who has always supported me.

I thank Caroline, my sister, for her wise counsel.

And to my friend Florence who encouraged me throughout the writing of this book.

Finally

Our thanks to Odile Jacob and Caroline Rolland, our editors, in whom we found support and good advice that helped us bring this book to fruition.

Profound thanks are due to medical herbalist Julian Barker for his expert translation of this book. Julian is especially well suited to this task, since, in addition to being conversant with both the English and French languages, he has studied Endobiogeny for many years, first with Dr. Duraffourd and myself, and later with Dr. Kamyar Hedayat. His accuracy, fluency, and intimacy with the subtleties and nuances of Endobiogeny are particularly prized. His work is particularly valuable in that this is the first book in English on Endobiogeny that is aimed at both the general public and medical practitioners.

NOTES

Introduction

1. Rimonabant is a medication developed by the French pharmaceutical company Sanofi Aventis for management of obesity and elevated cholesterol. It was approved in 2006 by the European Union and removed from the market by 2008 on account of its serious psychiatric side effects including suicide. The US Food and Drug Administration never approved it for sale.

2. Benfluorex is another obesity drug developed by the French company Servier. It was on the market for 33 years (1976–2009). It was linked to the deaths of 500–1,000 people from heart failure resulting from damage to a heart valve.

3. Rofecoxib is a medication developed by Merck for management of arthritis-related pain. After being on the market for 15 years (1999–2004), it was voluntarily withdrawn when research demonstrated that it was associated with heart attacks, many of them fatal. In the US alone it was estimated that over 100,000 heart attacks with 30,000–40,000 of them fatal occurred as a result. Merck has paid nearly $1 billion in fines and settlements over this one drug. It was also discovered that the company knew their drug was harmful and withheld this information for years.

4. Between 2000 and 2004, 8,473 new cases of cancers have been recorded in children less than 15 years of age.
5. The Nutrition Institute of America, http://www.stopcancer.com/medical-mistakes.htm, and http://www.angelfire.com/az/sthurston/Leading_Cause_of_ Death_in_the_US.html
6. Since the publication of this book in 2012, overseas interest has continued to grow, including Lithuania, Great Britain, and Canada.

Chapter one

1. The Opposable Medical References (RMO) are recommendations of good medical practices concerning a pathology rather than particular clinical cases. Created in order to avoid harmful prescriptions, they are not mandatory although enforceable in daily medical practice.
2. According to the official definition, consensus conferences are "standardized methods of scientific conduct of a process of collective reflection intended for discussing controversial issues raised by legitimate authority and imposing public recommendations."
3. *Docteur Nature*, Fayard press, 1971.
4. It is referred to as "Clinical Phytotherapy" because the selection of medicinal plants (Phytotherapy) is determined not solely by the patient's symptoms but by the global clinical picture as diagnosed by the physician.
5. Terrain-based medicine is a medicine based in modern scientific concepts of physiology. In our system, "terrain" refers to all the structural elements of a person such as their cells, tissues, organs, circulatory channels, etc. and their functional elements: how these structural parts function on their own and in conjunction with other parts and systems, such as the endocrine, nervous and immune systems.
6. Levothyroxine is a synthetic version of the thyroid hormone thyroxine (T_4). Commercial names include Synthroid®, Levoxyl® and Unithyroid®.
7. French Agency for the Safety of Health Products (AFSSA), renamed National Agency for the Safety of Medicines and Health Products (MSNA) in July, 2011.
8. Endogenous aggressors include genetics and the specific expression of the genetic potential (phenotype) at various phases of life, seasons, times of the day, etc. We often restrict our thinking about genetic factors to people with have dysfunctional enzymes or receptors, with a lack or an excess of certain hormones or immune factors, etc. There are,

however, subtle genetic variations, for example, the tendency to have a sweet tooth, or to have a liver with either a more compromised or a larger capacity than average. Finally, in the interaction of the exogenous and endogenous factors we have epigenetic factors, which modify our genetic potential.

9. Such as those responsible for issuing marketing authorizations, or assessing the quality of essential oils.

10. Roughly equivalent to €25 today.

11. Discussed in further detail in Chapter 8 "Debate Around the Diseases of Civilization."

12. As of 2016, the expert system is used in the United States, Canada, Mexico, Great Britain, France, Belgium, Lithuania, and Tunisia. The number of specialists has also grown to include gastroenterologists, endocrinologists, obstetricians-gynecologists, cardiologists, pediatricians, functional dentists, and many others.

Chapter two

1. François Jacob (born 1920 in Nancy), Jacques Lucien Monod (born 1910 in Paris, died 1976 in Cannes) and André Lwoff (born 1902 in Ainay-le-Château, died in Paris 1994) developed the gene operon theory and were awarded the Nobel Prize in Physiology & Medicine in 1965 for their discoveries of the genetic control of enzyme synthesis and viral replication.

2. Cited in the article "Human Genome: The Hour of Disillusionment," *Courrier International* (French weekly newspaper), June, 2010.

3. These SNP (single nucleotide polymorphism) techniques are based on the DNA variation between individuals of the same species in which two chromosomes differ in a given segment by the identity of a single base pair.

4. If, in general, the genes and the environment will contribute to shape the state of an individual, a gene predisposing to a disease will not, in itself, cause the disease, although its presence increases the risk for the individual to develop it.

5. See http://www.sante.gouv.fr/IMG/pdf/EMIR.pdf

6. Therapy aimed at introducing in a patient the normal copy of the gene or defective genes responsible for the disease that one wishes to cure, or to cause a change in their expression.

7. The use of a retroviral vector consists in introducing in a patient the normal copy of the defective gene(s) responsible for the disease that one wishes to cure, or to cause a change in their expression.

8. EMBO Reports, 2007, 8, p. 429–432.

9. European Molecular Biology Organization (EMBO).

10. http://www.inserm.fr/content/download/10200/76098/version/1/file/therapie_genique_esperances.pdf

11. David L. Sackett et coll., "Evidence based medicine: What it is and what it isn't," *BMJ*, 1996, p. 312, doi: 10.1136/bmj.312.7023.71.

12. A randomized controlled trial is a study of the effects of a treatment during which the subjects are randomly distributed into a control group and an experimental group.

13. In this type of study, the subjects are divided into two groups chosen randomly and entirely by chance, and neither the patient nor the doctor knows if they take no treatment (a placebo-controlled study) or a previously tested treatment (a positive-control study).

14. This is a major annual Medical & Pharmaceutical Trade Show that brings together thousands of professionals.

15. Médiator is a weight loss drug in the same family as the infamous Fen-phen and related to amphetamines.

16. http://www.armees.com/IMG/pdf/liste_des_77_medicaments_sous_surveillance.pdf

17. http://sante.journaldesfemmes.com/maux-quotidien/retrait-marche-actos-et-competact-0611.shtml

18. http://www.atoute.org/n/article203.htm

19. Upstene has been associated with potentially serious birth defects of the head, heart, and abdomen.

20. We read with interest the work of Gilbert Chauvet, *Comprendre l'organisation du vivant et son évolution vers la conscience* (English: *Understanding the Organization of Living Beings and the Evolution Toward Consciousness*), Paris, Vuibert; Collection *Automates Intelligents* (English: *Intelligent Automata*), February, 2006.

Chapter three

1. For any information concerning the teaching organized by the International Society of Endobiogenic Medicine and Integrative Physiology (SIMEPI, a non-profit association, law of 1901), please refer to http://www.simepi.info/spip.php?heading7; United States: http://www.endobiogeny.com

2. In French, the term "biology" refers to the biomarkers tested from blood or other body fluid samples. The term "function" is referring to the functional activity of the body. Not the potential for action but what has actually happened, how the body is functioning in real time. Thus, the term "Biology of Functions" means "functional biomarker analysis."
3. Pathogenecity is the specific genetic tendency for a person to express disease in a particular organ or with an imbalance along certain hormonal lines.
4. Ricardo Vélez, "Une sylviculture anti-incendie" (English: Preventing Forest Fires Through Silviculture), *FAO Documents Archive*, 1990, No. 162.
5. For more details, please refer to the Bibliography at the end of the book.
6. These are the last small ramifications of the bronchi ensuring the access of air to the alveoli of the lung, where gas exchange with the blood takes place.
7. Of course, one should consider the differences in climate and inversion of seasons, depending on whether the person lives in the northern or southern hemisphere.
8. Pierre Lapraz, *Étude biologique et clinique de l'aromathérapie et discussion de son intérêt* (English: *Biological and Clinical Study of Aromatherapy and Related Discussions*, thesis in medicine), François-Rabelais University, Tours, 1979.

Chapter four

1. See Chapter 5: "What Type of Terrain Are You?"
2. The thyroid exerts a specific action on the metabolism, on the tissues, on the brain, on behavior, on memory.
3. Studies currently underway:

   – assessment of the risk of mortality in patients with cancers based on certain Biology of Functions indexes. In collaboration with researchers from Scripps Research Institute (USC, University of South California);
   – assessment of the survival rate in children under intensive palliative based on certain Biology of Functions indexes. Children Memorial Hospital of Chicago, and researchers of the Northwestern University (Chicago).

4. See the Bibliography at the end of this book.

Chapter five

1. As confirmed by modern genetics even for identical (monozygotic) twins.
2. These tables are presented so as to give the reader some general ideas. In no way are they designed for self-diagnosis nor to substitute for the personal care of a qualified physician.
3. David Servan-Schreiber, *Guérir le stress, l'anxiété et la dépression sans médicaments ni psychanalyse* (English: *Healing Stress, Anxiety and Depression Without Medication or Psychoanalysis*), Paris, Robert Laffont, 2003.
4. This detached libido corresponds with Aristotle's observation *"Post coitum, omne animale triste."*

Chapter six

1. The Evin Law of 1989 completely discredited plant-based magistral preparations (medicinal product prepared in a pharmacy in accordance with a medical prescription for an individual patient) by refusing their refund.
2. At the time Doctor Valnet raised public awareness of medicinal plants with his best-seller *Docteur nature* (English: *Doctor Nature*), Paris, Fayard, 1971.
3. By interacting with the Cytochrome P450 3A4 (abbreviated CYP3A4).
4. Measures the clotting time of a subject under anticoagulant treatment compared to a normal subject. The lower the number, the greater is the risk of thrombosis (blood clot).
5. *MediaDico.*
6. See the Press Release: "Inauguration of a Center Specialized in Integrative Medicine in Mexico City: 45 medical doctors trained in Clinical Phytotherapy by the SIMEPI," http://www.simepi.info/spip.php?article20
7. Julian Barker, *History, Philosophy and Medicine: Phytotherapy in Context*, Winter Press, 2007.
8. Alan G. Morton, *History of Botanical Science*, London, Academic Press, 1981.
9. Susan P. Mattern, *The Prince of Medicine: Galen in the Roman Empire*, Oxford, Oxford University Press, 2013.
10. Morton *op cit* p. 89.

11. C. Duraffourd and J.-C. Lapraz, *La phytothérapie: retour vers le futur* (English: *Phytotherapy: Back to the Future*), December, 1994.
12. Whole extracts are substances made by extracting a vegetable substance by using a solvent such as water, alcohol, oil.
13. These are galenic formulations with international patents pending in the United States, Europe and China. Without the need for preservatives, microspheres assure great stability of the active principles over a wide range of climatic conditions.
14. Conducted by Professor Aliou Balde, Director of the Center for Research and Exploitation of Medicinal Plants of Kopere (CRVPM Dubréka, Guinea Conakry) and Dr. Sohar Traoré, in collaboration with the pharmaceutical laboratory AMB Pharma (Guinea) and the pharmaceutical group Michel Iderne (France).

Chapter seven

1. Doctors F. Alliot, A. Brisard, A. Carillon, M. Charles, A. Crochard, David-Henriau, T. Desgranges, R. Dodeur, H. Fontaine, M.-T. Gourdier, G. Grimaldi, M. Guyader, M. Henriot, J. Loubet, P. Lapraz, S. Michel, M.-O. Renaudin, J.-P. Renault, H. Roduit, T. Telphon.
2. C. Duraffourd, J.-C. Lapraz with contributions from R. Chemli, *La Plante médicinale, de la tradition à la science* (English: *Medicinal Plant, from Tradition to Science*), Paris, Éditions Jacques Grancher, 1997.
3. Doctor of Osteopathy.
4. Certified Nutritionist.
5. Endobiogenic Integrative Medical Center (EIMC).
6. President and founding member, American Society of Endobiogenic Medicine and Integrative Physiology, Vice-President, International Federation of Endobiogenic Medicine and Integrative Physiology (FIMEPI).
7. Dr. Hedayat was chief of pediatric intensive care and integrative medicine in Shreveport, Louisiana prior to studying Endobiogeny.
8. Dopamine is a neurotransmitter that increases focus and decision-making capabilities.
9. Program leader, BSc Herbal Medicine (Phytotherapy), London, Middlesex University.
10. Member of the BEMS, English Society of Endobiogenic Medicine.
11. *ibid.*

12. Gross enlargement of a limb due to blockage in the lymphatic vessels leading to a massive lymph-edema.
13. Paul Hersch Martínez, Doctor of Medicine and Social Sciences and Health, Member of the National Academy of Pharmaceutical Sciences (ANCF), researcher at the National Institute of Anthropology and History (INAH), President of the Sociedad Mexicana de Fitoterapia Clinica (SMFC) (English-Mexican Society of Clinical Phytotherapy) (Somefic), Member of the National Society of Researchers (SNI), of the Permanent Commission on Pharmacopoeia and of the IUCN Medicinal Plants Conservation Commission.
14. *Gaceta Oficial del Distrito Federal*, "Decreto por el que se expide the Ley de salud del Distrito Federal" (English: *Official Gazette of the Federal District*, Decree on the Health Law of the Federal District), Gaceta Oficial del Distrito Federal, September 17, 2009, 677, p. 5.
15. Head of the Department of Phytotherapy at the Center of Integrative Medicine (CEMI, Department of Health, Mexico City), Secretary General of the Mexican Society of Clinical Phytotherapy (SOMEFIC).
16. Member of the Mexican Society of Clinical Phytotherapy (SOMEFIC).
17. P. Chasseuil and J.-C. Charrié, "Le centre hospitalier de La Rochelle met le cap sur la cicatrisation; une vision intégrative de la prise en charge des plaies avec le Centre d'activité plaies et cicatrisation (CAPCic)" (English: The Hospital Center of La Rochelle Has the Answer for Healing; an Integrative View on the Management of Wounds with Center for Wound Healing (CAPCic)), *Journal des plaies et cicatrisation* (*Journal of Wound Care*), September, 2010, No. 75, tome XV.
18. Dr. J.-C. Charrié, *ABC de l'argile* (English, ABC of the Clay), Paris, Editions Grancher, 2007.
19. Heading "Colloques et manifestations" (English: Conferences and Various Events) at http://www.simepi.info/spip.php?article13
20. National WHO Program against leprosy, Department of Major Endemic Disease of the Ministry of Health.
21. She had 4 g/L in her blood against a desirable level of 2.40 g/L, or even 2 g/L in high-risk cases.
22. A drug that contains iodine and consequently may cause an iodine overload.
23. TSH at 0.02 as compared with a normal level of 2–4; T4 at 2.85 as compared with a normal level between 0.70 and 1.90; T3 at 6.7 as compared with a normal level between 3.4 and 7.2.

24. An autoimmune disease in which antibody against elements of the thyroid gland become highly positive.

25. Biological assessment: TSH at 220 (normal level < 4); the peripheral thyroid hormones T3 and T4 cannot be detected.

Chapter eight

1. National Health and Nutrition Examination Survey.

2. http://www.medscape.org/viewprogram/32094

3. Frank W. Pfrieger and Thomas Claudepierre (Neurochemistry Center of Strasbourg) et al., "CNS Synaptogenesis Promoted by Glia-Derived Cholesterol," *Science*, 2001, 294 (5545), pp. 1354–1357.

4. These fundamental reactions control oxidation and anti-oxidative activity in cells and tissues.

5. Readers might like to refer back to Chapter 3 "A True Terrain-Based Medicine."

6. Framingham Heart Study, 1948.

7. Heart Protection Study on Simvastatin (Zocor®).

8. Marketed under several names: Lipitor®, Tahor® (€109.24 per box containing 90, 80 mg tablets) produced by Pfizer (U.S.), Astellas (Japan), and Almirall (Spain).

9. A generic drug is one that contains the same active ingredient(s) as the named brand drug, but with a different presentation and excipients, and comes in at a lower price.

10. Crestor®, €103.80 per box containing 90, 20 mg tablets.

11. Befizal®, Ciprofibrate®, Fegenor®, Fenofibrate®, Lipanor®, Lipanthyl®, Lipur®, Secalip®.

12. The fibrates are activators of PPAR-alpha (peroxisome proliferator-activated receptors alpha).

13. Abbott, Actavis, Alter, Arrow Génériques, Biogaran, Cristers, EG labo, Fournier, Hexal Biotech, Leurquin Mediolanum, Mylan, Pfizer, Qualimed, Ranbaxy, Ratiopharm, Sandoz, Sanofi Aventis, Téva Santé, Zydus France.

14. A process that causes massive destruction of muscle fibers with a drop in calcium and an increase in potassium levels in the blood, with serious, even fatal consequences.

15. http://www.ncbi.nlm.nih.gov/pubmed/8283157

16. Gemfibrozil, marketed since 1982 as Lipur® by Pfizer Laboratory.

17. The process of deposition of fatty acids and cholesterol plaques on the walls of arteries.

18. In France, four molecules belonging to the class of fibrates have national marketing authorization: bezafibrate (Befizal® authorized since 1982, Actavis Group PTC), ciprofibrate (Lipanor® authorized since 1983, Sanofi Aventis laboratory + generics), fenofibrate (Lipanthyl®, authorized since 1986, Fournier laboratory + generics; Fenocor® authorized since 1987, Leurquin Mediolanum laboratory + generics), and gemfibrozil (Lipur® authorized since 1982, Pfizer laboratory).

19. Sold under the brand names Cholstat®, Staltor®, Baycol®, Lipobay®.

20. Michel de Lorgeril, *Cholestérol, mensonges et propagande* (English: *Cholesterol, Lies and Propaganda*), Vergèze, Editions Thierry Souccar, 1998.

21. Study of the side effects of drugs.

22. Application of epidemiological methods to evaluate the effects of drugs, be they beneficial or undesirable.

23. Marc Girard, Alertes grippales (Flu Alerts). *Comprendre et choisir* (English: *Understanding and choosing*), Escalquens, Editions Dangles, 2009; and the same author, and same editor, *Médicaments dangereux, à qui la faute?* (English: *Harmful Drugs, Who's to Be Blamed?*), 2011.

24. American study on 41,000 patients, published in July, 2007, A. A. Alsheikh-Ali, P. V. Maddukuri, Hui Han, R. H. Karas, "Effect of the magnitude of lipid lowering on risk of elevated liver enzymes, rhabdomyolysis, and cancer: Insights from large randomized statin trials," *Journal of American College of Cardiology*, 2007, 50 (5) 409–418.

25. "Low serum cholesterol level and attempted suicide," *American Journal of Psychiatry*, 1995, 152, 419–423.

26. For example, in the case of inherited autosomal dominant disorder with monogenic homozygous familial hypercholesterolemia.

27. As described in Chapter 4 "Behind the Closed Doors of the Exam Room."

28. Such we saw in the case of Marie-Laure in Chapter 4.

29. Reimbursement data from the Assurance Maladie (SNIIRAM, CnamTS, 2007).

30. C. Cornu et al., "Effect of intensive glucose lowering treatment on all cause mortality, cardiovascular death, and microvascular events in type 2 diabetes: Meta-analysis of randomized controlled trials," *BMJ*, 2011, 343, p. d4169.

31. Even if the risk of nonfatal myocardial infarction was slightly reduced (by 15%), and that of micro-albuminuria (by 10%), an increase of 100% in the frequency of severe hypoglycemia was observed.

32. Zinman B, et coll. (Department of Medicine, Mount Sinai Hospital and University of Toronto, Canada), "Low-dose combination therapy with rosiglitazone and metformin to prevent type 2 diabetes mellitus CANOE trial: A double-blind randomised controlled studio," *Lancet*, 2010, 376 (9735), p. 103–111. And http://www.ncbi.nlm.nih.gov/pubmed/20605202

33. *The Lancet* is a British scientific journal recognized as the world leader in medical journals in the field of general medicine, oncology, neurology, and infectious diseases.

34. http://www.afssaps.fr/Infos-de-securite/Points-d-information/Medicaments-Avandia-et-Avandamet-retrait-du-marche-Point-d-information

35. Numerous mechanisms are involved: they block the natural hormones receptors and modulate their synthesis, their transport, their metabolism, and their excretion.

36. See the Appendix "Endocrine Disrupters" at the end of the book.

37. The French Parliamentary Office for Evaluation of Scientific and Technological Options (OPECST) approved on July 13, 2011 the report presented by Senator Gilbert Barbier on endocrine disrupters.

38. http://www.liberation.fr/societe/01012306988-il-y-a-des-confusions-d-interets-qui-choquent

Chapter ten

1. Projections from statistical modeling of disease incidence data reported in the cancer registry up until 2005, as well as national data on mortality due to cancer up until 2007.

2. Cancer prevalence in France in 2009, National Institute of Cancer.

3. See Chapter 8, "Debate Around the Diseases of Civilization."

4. The long-term illnesses (LTI) are diseases whose severity and chronicity require a prolonged treatment and particularly expensive therapeutic and no copayment.

5. According to the INCa (National Cancer Institute) report on the situation of chemotherapy in France in 2010: "The number of patients treated

by chemotherapy has increased by more than 24% compared with 2005. For the second consecutive year, the expenditure on so-called biotherapy molecules makes up the largest portion of the cost and represents 57% of the cost of all anticancer treatments."

6. Avastin of Roche Laboratory humanized monoclonal antibody that targets angiogenesis, the process of new blood vessel formation favoring the growth of tumors. The price of a 16 ml vial, €1,280, is 100% covered by the Social Security system of France.

7. FDA is the abbreviation for Food and Drug Administration, the US government agency responsible for the control and licensing of drugs prior to sale.

8. http://pharmacritique.20minutes-blogs.fr/avastin-enbrel-anticorps-mono-clonaux-anti-tnf/ and http://pharmacritique.20minutes-blogs.fr/archive/2010/12/23/avastin-n'est-plus-autorise-dans-le-cancer-du-sein-etats-uni.html

9. Phase 3 evaluates the clinical benefit of a new compound compared to a placebo or to another medicinal product.

10. Algeta Bayer press release of August 25, 2011, at the ASCO, reported by Guy Macy. http://www.pharmactua.com/tag/bayer/

11. The sequencing of genes of our species was completed in April, 2003 (Human Genome Project—HGP).

12. €2,500 per 30 tablets box, a cost that is 100% covered by the French Social Security system.

13. The gene encoding this protein located on the surface of cells whose increase promotes the growth of cancer cells is a proto-oncogene commonly called Her-2/neu.

14. Estrogen and Cytochrome P450 1B1 "Contribute to Both Early and Late-Stage Head and Neck Carcinogenesis," *Cancer Prev Res*, 2011, 4(1), p. 107–115.

15. Care for women at risk, RPC, Saint Paul de Vence, October, 2007.

16. Of the Centre de recherche sur les pathologies prostatiques in Paris.

17. "Médecines traditionnelles et cancers en Chine" (English: Traditional Medicines and Cancers in China), article published in the *Concours médical* of July 9, 1994.

18. Claude Bernard (1813–1878), *Introduction à l'étude de la médecine expérimentale* (English: *Introduction to the Study of Experimental Medicine*), Paris, Champs-Flammarion.

19. Jules Henri Poincaré (1854–1912) Mathematician who inaugurated the study of dynamical systems in the modern sense and wrote much about the philosophy of the scientific method.

Conclusion

1. Rozenn Dodeur, *Place des moyens thérapeutiques d'extraction naturelle pour les malades en soins palliatifs* (English: *The Place of Natural-Based Therapeutic Means for the Sick under Palliative Care*), Dissertation for the university diploma of palliative care, Lille Catholic University, 1996.

Appendix one

1. http://www.lemonde.fr/societe/article/2011/04/05/le-distilbene-aurait-des-effets-sur-trois-generations_1503080_3224.html
2. For a list of drugs containing parabens, see AFMT, official website of the French Association of Thyroid Disease Sufferers (AFMT): http://www.asso-maladesthyroide.org/article.php?id=183
3. http://www.assemblee-nationale.fr/12/rapports/r3512.asp
4. reseau-environnement-sante.fr/wp.../veille_BPA_juil-sept-2011.pdf
5. www.greenfacts.org/fr/pcb/pcb-greenfacts.pdf
6. http://www.asef-asso.fr/index.php?option=com_content&view=article&id=367&Itemid=288
7. http://www.senat.fr/rap/l09-318/l09-318_mono.html
8. http://reseau-environnement-sante.fr/2010/11/03/ressources/bulletin-de-veille-scientifique-bpa-n%C2%B07-3/
9. Institut national de recherche agronomique (INRA—French National Institute for Agricultural Research), Toulouse, Daniel Zalko.
10. http://leruisseau.iguane.org/spip.php?article1500
11. http://www.safewater.org/PDFS/knowthefacts/frenchfactsheets/Polluant-sorganiquespersistants.pdf

INDEX

Printed in the USA
CPSIA information can be obtained
at www.ICGtesting.com
LVHW071155210924
791745LV00006B/33